The POTS Exercise Reconditioning Workbook

A 16-Week Program from Recumbent to Upright Activity with Daily Tracking Logs and Symptom Management Tools

Jessamine Ramona Stringer

The information provided in this book is designed to provide helpful information on the subjects discussed. This book is not meant to be used, nor should it be used, to diagnose or treat any medical condition. For diagnosis or treatment of any medical problem, consult your physician. The publisher and author are not responsible for any specific health needs that may require medical supervision and are not liable for any damages or negative consequences from any treatment, action, application, or preparation to any person reading or following the information in this book.

First Edition, 2026

ISBN: 978-1-923646-52-0

This workbook is intended for educational and informational purposes only. It is not intended as a substitute for professional medical advice, diagnosis, or treatment. Always seek the advice of your physician or other qualified health provider before beginning any exercise program, especially if you have Postural Orthostatic Tachycardia Syndrome or any other medical condition.

The exercise protocols described in this workbook are based on published medical research but must be implemented only with explicit approval from your healthcare provider. Individual results vary. Not all patients will experience the same degree of improvement. Some individuals may not be appropriate candidates for this program due to specific medical contraindications.

Stop exercise immediately and seek medical attention if you experience chest pain, severe dizziness, fainting, irregular heartbeat, or other concerning symptoms during or after exercise.

The names and scenarios depicted in this book are purely for illustrative purposes only. Any resemblance to actual persons, living or dead, or actual events is purely coincidental. All case examples represent composite illustrations based on typical clinical presentations rather than specific individuals.

References to specific equipment, products, or brands are provided for informational purposes only and do not constitute endorsement. The author and publisher receive no compensation from any manufacturers or retailers mentioned in this workbook.

Results from this exercise program vary by individual. Completion of the 16-week protocol does not guarantee specific outcomes. Success depends on multiple factors including baseline severity, consistency of implementation, concurrent treatments, comorbid conditions, and individual physiology. This program is a tool for symptom management, not a cure for POTS.

By using this workbook, you acknowledge that you have read and understood this disclaimer and agree to assume full responsibility for your health and safety.

Table of Contents

Introduction

If you have Postural Orthostatic Tachycardia Syndrome, someone has probably told you to exercise. Your doctor mentioned it. You read about it online. The research says it works. And yet here you are, still unable to exercise, still symptomatic, still searching for something that actually helps.

The gap between "exercise helps POTS" and "I can successfully exercise with POTS" is massive. That gap is what this workbook addresses.

The Problem with Existing Resources

The research is clear. Studies by Levine, Fu, and others demonstrate that cardiovascular reconditioning improves POTS symptoms measurably. Heart size increases. Blood volume rises. Orthostatic intolerance decreases. The evidence is strong. The protocols exist.

What doesn't exist is a step-by-step workbook that takes you from unable to exercise to successfully reconditioned. The published protocols are PDFs meant for medical professionals, not patients trying to implement them alone. They assume access to exercise equipment, medical supervision, and the ability to follow complex instructions while symptomatic. Most POTS patients can't meet those assumptions.

General fitness programs don't work because they're designed for healthy people. They start upright. They progress too quickly. They don't account for post-exertional symptom exacerbation, orthostatic intolerance, or the unpredictability of autonomic dysfunction. Following a standard exercise program when you have POTS typically ends in crashes, discouragement, and abandonment.

You need something between the research protocols and general fitness advice. You need practical, day-by-day guidance written specifically for POTS reconditioning. That's what this workbook provides.

What Makes This Different

This workbook takes the evidence-based Levine and CHOP protocols and breaks them into manageable daily prescriptions. Every week has specific exercise prescriptions. Every session has duration, intensity, and position clearly defined. Every exercise includes form guidance and modifications. You know exactly what to do each day for 16 weeks.

The program starts with 3 minutes of recumbent exercise. Not 20 minutes. Not 30 minutes. Three minutes. Because that's where many POTS patients need to start. It builds by small increments that your deconditioned cardiovascular system can actually tolerate. It keeps you horizontal until your body is ready for upright work. It expects setbacks and provides protocols for managing them.

This is a workbook, not a book. The difference matters. You won't just read about exercise theory. You'll track every session. You'll record your heart rate, symptoms, and progress. You'll see objective data proving you're improving even when you feel like nothing is changing. The exercises built into each chapter ensure you're actively participating in your reconditioning, not passively consuming information.

Who This Is For

This workbook is for adults with diagnosed POTS who have medical clearance to exercise but struggle to do so successfully. It's for people who have tried to exercise and crashed. It's for those who can't follow standard protocols because the starting point is too advanced. It's for POTS patients who need structure, guidance, and proof that reconditioning is possible.

This program requires equipment. At minimum, you need access to a recumbent bike, supine pedaler, rowing machine, or pool. Upright exercise comes later, but you need recumbent options for the first eight weeks. The workbook provides alternatives and substitutions, but some equipment access is necessary.

This workbook is not for people with contraindications to exercise, those in acute medical crisis, or anyone without physician clearance. It's not a replacement for medical care. It's a tool to implement the exercise component of POTS management that your medical team has likely already recommended but hasn't given you practical guidance to execute.

What to Expect

This program takes 16 weeks if you follow it as prescribed. Some people need longer. That's fine. The timeline matters less than completing the progression. You'll move through four phases: Foundation, Building Endurance, Transitioning Upright, and Upright Mastery. Each phase has specific goals and builds on the previous one.

The first month is the hardest. You'll feel more fatigued. You'll question if this is working. You'll be tempted to quit. Most people who abandon the protocol do so in the first four weeks, right before the breakthrough happens. If you can push through Month 1, Month 2 brings genuine improvement. Month 3 shows undeniable progress. Month 4 confirms you've reconditioned your cardiovascular system.

You'll need to track consistently. The daily logs take two minutes post-exercise. The weekly reviews take five minutes. The monthly assessments take 10 minutes. This tracking isn't busy work. It's how you prove to yourself that the protocol is working when your subjective experience says otherwise.

You'll encounter problems. You'll crash at some point. You'll get sick. You'll have terrible days. Part 3 provides troubleshooting protocols for every common issue. Use them. Modify when necessary. Keep showing up. Consistency beats perfection.

The Evidence Base

This workbook adapts the Levine exercise protocol and the Children's Hospital of Philadelphia CHOP protocol, both supported by peer-reviewed research. Fu and Levine's 2018 study demonstrated that three months of exercise training increased heart mass, blood volume, and peak oxygen uptake in POTS patients. George et al. showed 90% of patients who completed a structured exercise program had significant symptom improvement. Shibata et al. documented measurable cardiac changes with sustained training.

The research shows this works. What the research doesn't show is how to actually do it when you're starting from severe deconditioning. That's what this workbook adds. It takes validated protocols and makes them executable for real patients with real limitations.

How to Use This Book

Read Part 1 first. All three chapters. Understand why exercise works, what you need before starting, and how to use the program. Don't skip to the workouts. The foundation matters.

Complete the baseline measurements in Chapter 2.0. You'll retake these every four weeks. The comparison data becomes your proof of progress.

Start Week 1 on a Monday. Follow the daily prescriptions exactly as written. Track every session. Complete the weekly reflections. Do the monthly assessments. The structure exists for a reason. Trust it.

Keep Part 3 accessible throughout the program. You'll reference the exercise library for form checks, the tracking systems for organization, and the troubleshooting chapter when problems arise. These are working tools, not supplementary reading.

After Week 16, use Chapter 7.0 to transition to maintenance. The reconditioning phase ends. The maintenance phase begins. Exercise becomes a permanent part of your POTS management, like medication and salt.

A Note on Realistic Expectations

This program will improve your POTS symptoms. It will increase your exercise capacity. It will expand what you can do in daily life. It will not cure you. POTS is a chronic condition. Exercise is a management tool, not a cure.

Some patients see dramatic improvement. They return to near-normal function. Others see moderate improvement. They can do significantly more than before but still have limitations. A few see minimal improvement and need to explore other treatment options. The research shows most people fall in the first two categories. You won't know until you complete the protocol.

What this program definitely will do is recondition your cardiovascular system. Your heart will be measurably larger. Your blood volume will be measurably higher. Your orthostatic heart rate increase will be measurably lower. These are objective, verifiable changes. Whether those changes translate to major symptom relief or moderate symptom relief varies by individual. Both outcomes are valuable.

Final Thoughts Before You Begin

You're about to do something difficult. Sixteen weeks of consistent exercise when exercise has been impossible is a significant undertaking. There will be days you want to quit. Days when you question if it's working. Days when lying in bed feels easier than getting on the bike.

On those days, remember this: thousands of POTS patients have completed this protocol before you. The majority succeeded. The ones who quit usually did so in the first four weeks, right before the progress became undeniable. If you can get through the first month, you can finish the program.

The data doesn't lie. If you show up consistently, track accurately, and follow the progression, your cardiovascular system will adapt. You'll see it in the numbers even when you can't feel it yet. Eventually, you'll feel it too.

You have the tools. You have the plan. You have the evidence that this works. Now you need 16 weeks of showing up. That's it. Just show up.

PART 1: UNDERSTANDING YOUR FOUNDATION

Chapter 1.0: Why Exercise Works for POTS

You already know exercise helps POTS. Your doctor told you. The support groups talk about it. You've read the articles. But here's is the thing: knowing exercise works and actually being able to do it are two completely different things. You've probably tried and felt worse. Maybe you pushed through and crashed for days. Maybe you gave up because it seemed impossible. It is possible your approach was wrong.

1.1 The Deconditioning Trap

Your heart is smaller than it should be. Not damaged—just smaller. Research shows POTS patients have reduced heart size and lower blood volume compared to healthy people. When your heart is smaller, it pumps less blood with each beat. To make up for this, it beats faster. Much faster. Especially when you stand up or try to move.

Here's the trap: POTS makes you feel terrible when you move, so you move less. When you move less, your heart gets even smaller. Your blood volume drops more. Your muscles weaken. Your symptoms get worse. Then moving feels even more impossible. This is the deconditioning cycle, and it's why you feel stuck.

Think of it like this: Your body adapted to being still. It got efficient at doing nothing. Now when you ask it to do something, it panics. Your heart races. You feel dizzy. You get exhausted. Your body isn't trying to hurt you—it's just confused about what you're asking it to do.

The good news? Hearts can grow. Blood volume can increase. Muscles can strengthen. But only if you recondition them the right way.

Exercise 1.1A: Recognize Your Pattern

This exercise helps you see how the deconditioning cycle shows up in your life.

Think about the last three months. Answer honestly—no one else needs to see this.

1. What activities have you stopped doing because of POTS symptoms?

____

____

____

2. What do you avoid now that you used to do regularly?

3. How has reducing activity affected your symptoms? (Got better? Stayed the same? Got worse?)

4. What would you do tomorrow if you knew exercise wouldn't make you crash?

1.2 Why Traditional Exercise Fails

You've tried to exercise. You followed advice from well-meaning people who don't have POTS. "Just start walking!" "Try yoga!" "Push through it!" And you crashed. Hard.

Traditional exercise advice fails POTS patients for one critical reason: it assumes your cardiovascular system works normally. It doesn't. When most people stand up and move, their body automatically sends blood to their brain. Your body struggles with this. When most people exercise upright, their heart rate increases appropriately. Yours skyrockets.

Standard exercise programs start with activities that require you to be upright—walking, jogging, standing exercises. For POTS patients, this is like asking someone with a broken leg to run a marathon. You're not being weak. You're not lacking willpower. You're being asked to do something your body genuinely cannot handle yet.

Here's what happens when you try standard exercise too soon: You stand up. Your blood pools in your legs. Your brain doesn't get enough blood. Your heart races trying to fix this. You feel dizzy, nauseous, exhausted. You push through because you're supposed to. Your body goes into crisis mode. You crash for days.

This isn't exercise intolerance. This is your body screaming that the approach is wrong.

Exercise 1.2A: Your Exercise History

This exercise helps you identify what went wrong with past attempts.

Think about times you've tried to exercise with POTS.

1. What types of exercise did you try?

---

2. What happened during the exercise? (Check all that apply)

[ ] Heart rate went extremely high (above 150-160)

[ ] Felt dizzy or lightheaded

[ ] Felt nauseous

[ ] Had to stop early

[ ] Felt okay during but terrible after

[ ] Nearly passed out

[ ] Chest pain or tightness

[ ] Extreme fatigue during

3. What happened in the 24-48 hours after exercise?

---

4. Looking back, what position were you in during these exercises? (Standing? Upright? Seated?)

1.3 What Makes This Protocol Different

This program works because it respects what your body actually needs: time, position, and progression.

Position matters: You start lying down or recumbent. Your heart doesn't have to fight gravity to get blood to your brain. You can actually exercise without triggering the cascade of POTS symptoms. This isn't cheating—this is strategic reconditioning.

Time matters: You start with 3-5 minutes. Not 30 minutes. Not even 10 minutes. Just a few minutes that your body can actually handle. Then you build one minute at a time. This is slow by normal standards. But POTS isn't normal, and rushing is what made you crash before.

Progression matters: You stay horizontal for weeks, sometimes months. You build endurance while recumbent. Only when your body is genuinely ready do you transition to upright exercise. You earn each progression by proving your body can handle the current level.

The CHOP Protocol and Levine Protocol both follow this approach. They were specifically designed for POTS patients based on years of research. They work because they meet your body where it actually is, not where you wish it was.

Exercise 1.3A: Understanding Your Starting Point

This exercise helps you see why starting horizontal makes sense for you.

Rate your symptoms on a scale of 1-10 (1 = no problem, 10 = severe) for each position:

Position	Heart Rate Response	Dizziness	Fatigue	Nausea
Lying down	____	____	____	____
Sitting	____	____	____	____
Standing still	____	____	____	____
Walking	____	____	____	____

What do you notice about your symptoms as you move from horizontal to upright?

____

____

____

Why does starting with recumbent exercise make sense for your body?

____

____

____

1.4 The Science That Supports You

Dr. Benjamin Levine's research team studied POTS patients for years. They discovered that structured exercise training increases heart size, expands blood volume, and improves how much oxygen your body can use. Patients who completed the exercise protocol showed measurable improvements in heart function and symptom reduction.

One study followed POTS patients through three months of training. Their hearts grew larger. Their blood volume increased. Their peak oxygen uptake improved by 11%. Their heart rate during activity decreased because their hearts pumped more efficiently. Most importantly, their quality of life improved significantly.

This isn't about pushing through or building mental toughness. This is about physically changing your cardiovascular system. Your heart can literally grow. Your blood vessels can work better. Your muscles can help pump blood back to your heart. These are measurable, physical changes that happen when you recondition correctly.

Research shows this protocol works for about 90% of POTS patients who stick with it. The key phrase: stick with it. Most people who quit do so in the first month, before the real changes happen.

Exercise 1.4A: Connect to the Evidence

This exercise helps you understand what exercise can actually change for you.

Based on the research, what physical changes can happen with this protocol?

____

____

____

Which of these changes would make the biggest difference in your daily life?

____

____

____

On a scale of 1-10, how much do you believe this protocol could work for you?

1 _____ 2 _____ 3 _____ 4 _____ 5 _____ 6 _____ 7 _____ 8 _____ 9 _____ 10

What makes you uncertain? (It's okay to have doubts)

1.5 The First Month Paradox

Here's what nobody warns you about: the first month might make you feel worse, not better. Your fatigue may increase. You might feel more tired than usual. This doesn't mean it's not working—it means it IS working.

Your body is being asked to do something it's not used to doing. Even lying down and pedaling for 5 minutes is work when you're deconditioned. Your muscles are waking up. Your cardiovascular system is being challenged. This creates fatigue. Legitimate, real fatigue.

This is not the crash you experienced with traditional exercise. This is the fatigue of adaptation. It's temporary. It's expected. It's actually a sign your body is responding.

Most people who quit do so in Month 1. They feel worse and assume the protocol isn't working. They give up right before the breakthrough happens. Month 2 is when most people start feeling genuinely better. Month 3 is when the improvements become undeniable.

Your job in Month 1 is simple: keep showing up. Do the work. Accept the fatigue. Trust that your body is changing even when you can't feel it yet. The people who succeed are the ones who keep going when it's hard.

Exercise 1.5A: Prepare for Reality

This exercise helps you set realistic expectations and plan for the hard parts.

Week 1-4 Expectations: What might you experience? (Check all you understand are normal)

[ ] Increased fatigue

[ ] Feeling more tired than usual

[ ] Wondering if this is working

[ ] Wanting to quit

[ ] Not seeing immediate improvements

[ ] Feeling discouraged

[ ] Muscle soreness

What will you tell yourself when you feel worse in Week 2?

____

____

____

Who can support you during the hard first month?

Name: ____

How they'll help: ____

____

What will be your sign to keep going even when it's hard?

____

____

____

1.6 Your Commitment to Change

This protocol works. But only if you work it. You need to commit to 16 weeks of consistent effort. Not perfect effort—consistent effort. You'll have bad days. You'll miss sessions. That's normal. What matters is that you keep coming back.

You're not committing to feeling better immediately. You're committing to showing up and doing the work. The results will come. Your heart will grow. Your blood volume will increase. Your symptoms will improve. But first, you have to prove to your body that you're serious about this change.

Exercise 1.6A: Make Your Commitment

This exercise helps you commit to the full 16 weeks before you start.

Complete this commitment statement:

I, ________________________________, commit to following this exercise protocol for 16 weeks.

I understand that:

- The first month may be difficult
- I might feel worse before I feel better
- Changes take time to appear
- Consistency matters more than perfection
- Missing a few sessions doesn't mean failure

I'm doing this because:

____

____

____

When I want to quit, I'll remember:

____

____

____

My start date will be: ____________________

My Week 16 completion date will be: ____________________

Signature: ____________________________________ **Date:** ____________________

1.7 Chapter at a Glance

- Your heart is smaller and your blood volume is lower because of POTS—this is the deconditioning cycle
- Traditional exercise fails because it starts upright when your body can't handle that yet
- This protocol works by starting horizontal, building slowly, and progressing only when ready
- Research shows exercise increases heart size, blood volume, and oxygen capacity in POTS patients
- The first month will be hard and you might feel worse—this is normal and temporary
- Commitment to the full 16 weeks is required for real results
- About 90% of people who complete the protocol see significant improvement

Chapter 2.0: Before You Begin

You're ready to start. You understand why this works. You're committed. But jumping straight into exercise without preparation is a mistake that leads to crashes and discouragement. This chapter ensures you have everything in place before Day 1. Do not skip this preparation work. It's the foundation that makes everything else possible.

2.1 Medical Clearance Essentials

Before starting any exercise program with POTS, you need to talk with your doctor. Not because exercise is dangerous, but because your specific situation might require modifications. Some people have additional cardiac issues. Some take medications that affect heart rate. Some have comorbidities that change the approach.

Your doctor needs to know you're starting this program. They can review your medications, check for any cardiac issues that need monitoring, and confirm you're safe to begin. If you're working with a cardiologist or dysautonomia specialist, even better. They understand POTS exercise protocols.

Bring this workbook to your appointment. Show them the program structure. Most doctors familiar with POTS will recognize the CHOP/Levine approach and support it. If your doctor says "don't exercise," ask specifically about recumbent exercise. The research is clear—this helps POTS. If they're unfamiliar with POTS exercise protocols, you might need to educate them or seek a second opinion from a dysautonomia specialist.

Exercise 2.1A: Medical Clearance Checklist

This exercise ensures you've covered all necessary medical bases before starting.

Complete this checklist before beginning the program:

[ ] Scheduled appointment with my doctor/cardiologist

[ ] Discussed starting this exercise program with my healthcare provider

[ ] Reviewed my current medications and how they might affect exercise

[ ] Confirmed no cardiac issues that would prevent exercise

[ ] Asked about any specific modifications I need

[ ] Got clearance to begin (or scheduled follow-up if needed)

Doctor's name:

____

Date of clearance: ____________________

Specific instructions or modifications from my doctor:

____

____

____

Medications that might affect my heart rate during exercise:

____

____

Any concerns my doctor raised that I need to monitor:

____

____

____

2.2 Establishing Your Baseline

You need to know where you're starting so you can track progress. These baseline measurements will show you how much you're improving, even when it doesn't feel like it yet.

Take these measurements at the same time of day, ideally in the morning before eating or drinking caffeine. Wear comfortable clothing. Make sure you're well-hydrated before testing.

Lying Heart Rate and Blood Pressure: Lie flat for 5 minutes. Completely relax. Then measure your heart rate and blood pressure while still lying down. Record the numbers.

Standing Heart Rate and Blood Pressure: From lying position, stand up. Within 30 seconds to 1 minute, measure your heart rate and blood pressure. Stay standing but still. Take another measurement at 3 minutes. Take a final measurement at 5 minutes if you can tolerate standing that long.

These numbers tell you how much your heart rate increases when you stand (orthostatic intolerance). They also show how long you can comfortably stand. As you progress through the program, these numbers will improve. Your standing heart rate will be lower. You'll tolerate standing longer. But you need baseline data to see the change.

Exercise 2.2A: Record Your Baseline

This exercise captures your starting point for comparison later.

Date of baseline testing: ____________________

Time of day: ____________________

Lying Down Measurements (after 5 minutes rest):

Heart Rate: _____ bpm

Blood Pressure: _____ / _____ mmHg

How I felt:

____

Standing Measurements:

Time Point	Heart Rate	Blood Pressure	Symptoms
30 seconds after standing	_____ bpm	_____ / _____	_____________
3 minutes standing	_____ bpm	_____ / _____	_____________
5 minutes standing	_____ bpm	_____ / _____	_____________

Increase from lying to standing:

Heart Rate increase: _____ bpm (standing HR minus lying HR)

How long could you comfortably stand? ____________________

Other observations:

____

____

____

Note: You'll repeat these measurements at Week 4, Week 8, Week 12, and Week 16 to track improvement.

2.3 Calculating Your Heart Rate Zones

Heart rate zones tell you how hard you're working. Too easy and you won't recondition. Too hard and you'll crash. The zones keep you in the safe, effective range.

First, calculate your maximum heart rate: 220 minus your age = max HR.

Example: If you're 25 years old, 220 - 25 = 195 max HR.

Your training zones are percentages of this maximum:

Recovery Zone (50-60% max HR): Very easy, can talk normally, barely feels like exercise. Used for recovery days and when first starting.

Base Pace Zone (60-70% max HR): Comfortable but working, can still hold conversation, sustainable for long periods. Your primary training zone for Weeks 1-8.

Maximal Steady State (70-80% max HR): Working hard but sustainable, conversation gets harder, feels challenging. Used in Weeks 9-16.

Interval Zone (80-90% max HR): Hard work, can only say a few words, can't sustain long. Used briefly in advanced weeks.

Calculate each zone now. These will guide your entire program.

Exercise 2.3A: Calculate Your Zones

This exercise determines your personal heart rate training zones.

Step 1: Find Your Maximum Heart Rate

My age: _____ years

220 - _____ (age) = _____ (maximum heart rate)

Step 2: Calculate Each Zone

Recovery Zone (50-60% of max):

Max HR _____ × 0.50 = _____ (lower limit)

Max HR _____ × 0.60 = _____ (upper limit)

My Recovery Zone: _____ to _____ bpm

Base Pace Zone (60-70% of max):

Max HR _____ × 0.60 = _____ (lower limit)

Max HR _____ × 0.70 = _____ (upper limit)

My Base Pace Zone: _____ to _____ bpm

Maximal Steady State (70-80% of max):

Max HR _____ × 0.70 = _____ (lower limit)

Max HR _____ × 0.80 = _____ (upper limit)

My Maximal Steady State: _____ to _____ bpm

Interval Zone (80-90% of max):

Max HR _____ × 0.80 = _____ (lower limit)

Max HR _____ × 0.90 = _____ (upper limit)

My Interval Zone: _____ to _____ bpm

Write these numbers on a card you keep with your workout space. You'll reference them constantly.

2.4 RPE for Beta Blocker Users

If you take beta blockers (metoprolol, propranolol, atenolol, etc.), your heart rate won't respond normally to exercise. The medication prevents it from increasing much. This means you can't use heart rate zones to guide intensity. Instead, use the RPE (Rate of Perceived Exertion) scale.

RPE measures how hard the exercise feels to you, regardless of heart rate:

- **RPE 1-2**: Very easy, barely moving
- **RPE 3-4**: Light effort, comfortable, can talk easily (Recovery level)
- **RPE 5-6**: Moderate effort, working but comfortable, can talk in full sentences (Base Pace level)

- **RPE 7-8**: Hard effort, challenging, can only talk in short phrases (Maximal Steady State)
- **RPE 9-10**: Very hard, unsustainable for long, can barely talk (Interval level)

Your body knows when it's working hard. Trust that sensation. If the protocol says "Base Pace Zone," aim for RPE 5-6. If it says "Recovery," stay at RPE 3-4.

Exercise 2.4A: Understanding RPE

This exercise helps you learn to assess your effort level accurately.

For beta blocker users: Check here [ ] (I take beta blockers and will use RPE instead of heart rate)

My beta blocker medication:

____

Practice rating past activities:

Think about recent activities and estimate their RPE:

Activity	Estimated RPE (1-10)	Why I rated it this way
Sitting and reading	____	______________________________
Walking to bathroom	____	______________________________
Taking a shower	____	______________________________
Walking across parking lot	____	______________________________
Carrying groceries	____	______________________________

During exercise, I'll know I'm at the right intensity when:

RPE 3-4 (Recovery) feels like: ____

RPE 5-6 (Base Pace) feels like: ____

RPE 7-8 (Maximal Steady State) feels like:

____

2.5 Equipment and Setup

You don't need a gym membership or expensive equipment to start. You do need access to recumbent exercise options. Here are your choices:

Recumbent Bike (most common): Stationary bike where you sit back with legs extended forward. Can be found at gyms or purchased for home ($150-$500 for basic models).

Supine Pedaler (most affordable): Small pedal device you use while lying in bed or on floor. Very affordable ($30-$80). Good for starting.

Rowing Machine: Can be used seated. More expensive ($200-$800) but works whole body.

Swimming/Pool: Excellent option if you have access. Water supports your body and keeps you cool.

Resistance Bands: For strength training ($10-$20 for set). Essential for leg and core work.

Heart Rate Monitor: Chest strap or watch. Essential for non-beta-blocker users ($30-$200).

You need at least one recumbent cardio option and resistance bands. Everything else is optional. Start with what you can afford. You can add equipment as you progress.

Exercise 2.5A: Equipment Planning

This exercise helps you identify what equipment you have access to and what you need to acquire.

What I currently have access to:

[ ] Recumbent bike (location: ________________________________)

[ ] Supine pedaler

[ ] Rowing machine (location: ________________________________)

[ ] Pool for swimming (location: ________________________________)

[ ] Resistance bands

[ ] Heart rate monitor

[ ] Yoga mat or exercise mat

[ ] Other: ____

What I need to obtain before starting:

Item: ____________________________________ Estimated cost: _____ Plan to obtain by: __________

Item: ____________________________________ Estimated cost: _____ Plan to obtain by: __________

Item: ____________________________________ Estimated cost: _____ Plan to obtain by: __________

My budget for equipment: $ __________

Where I'll do cardio exercise: ____

Where I'll do strength training: ____

Backup options if my primary equipment isn't available:

____

____

____

2.6 Hydration and Salt Protocol

POTS patients need more salt and fluids than typical people. This isn't optional—it's essential for managing symptoms and enabling exercise. Dehydration makes everything worse. Low sodium makes exercise dangerous.

Daily baseline: Aim for 10-12 grams of sodium daily (check with your doctor, especially if you have high blood pressure or kidney issues). This is about 2-3 teaspoons of salt added to food throughout the day, plus salty foods.

Hydration target: 2-3 liters of fluids daily, more on exercise days. Water, electrolyte drinks, broth, sports drinks all count.

Before exercise: Drink 8-16 oz of fluid with electrolytes 30-60 minutes before exercising. This pre-loads your system.

During exercise: Keep water nearby. Sip every few minutes, especially if sweating.

After exercise: Drink 16-24 oz of fluid with sodium within 30 minutes of finishing. This prevents post-exercise crashes.

Salt loading before exercise significantly improves orthostatic tolerance. Some people take salt tablets (500-1000 mg) 30 minutes before exercise. Others drink electrolyte solutions. Find what works for you.

Exercise 2.6A: Create Your Hydration Plan

This exercise helps you establish your daily hydration and sodium protocol.

My doctor-approved daily sodium target: __________ grams (or __________ mg)

How I'll meet my sodium needs:

[ ] Adding salt to meals (approximately _____ teaspoons daily)

[ ] Salt tablets (_____ mg, _____ times daily)

[ ] Electrolyte drinks (brand: ________________________, _____ daily)

[ ] Salty foods (list: ____)

[ ] Broth or soup (_____ cups daily)

My daily fluid goal: __________ liters (or __________ ounces)

Before exercise:

What I'll drink:

____

How much: _____________________ When: _____________________

During exercise:

What I'll have available: ____

After exercise:

What I'll drink:

____

How much: ____________________ Within: ____________________ minutes

How I'll track my intake: (App? Water bottle marks? Journal?)

____

____

2.7 Compression Garments Guide

Compression stockings or leggings help prevent blood pooling in your legs. They can significantly reduce symptoms during and after exercise. Not everyone needs them, but many POTS patients benefit.

Compression levels: Measured in mmHg (millimeters of mercury):

- 15-20 mmHg: Light compression, good for mild symptoms
- 20-30 mmHg: Moderate compression, most commonly prescribed for POTS
- 30-40 mmHg: Firm compression, for severe symptoms (requires prescription)

Types: Knee-high, thigh-high, or full tights. Knee-high works for most people and is easier to put on.

When to wear: Put them on before standing up in morning. Wear during all upright activity and exercise. You can remove them when lying down for extended periods.

Getting them on: Harder than normal socks. Roll them up, slide foot in, gradually pull up. Easier when legs aren't already swollen.

Try compression for at least 2 weeks before deciding if it helps. Many people find it makes a significant difference in their ability to exercise.

Exercise 2.7A: Compression Assessment

This exercise helps you decide if you need compression garments and plan for obtaining them.

Do I currently use compression garments?

[ ] Yes, I already have compression (type: ________________, strength: _______ mmHg)

[ ] No, but I want to try them

[ ] No, I don't think I need them

[ ] I'm not sure if I should use them

If trying compression, my plan:

Compression level to try: __________ mmHg

Type: [ ] Knee-high [ ] Thigh-high [ ] Full tights

Where I'll obtain them: ____

Estimated cost: $ ___________

Questions to ask my doctor about compression:

____

____

____

When I'll wear them:

[ ] All day starting in morning

[ ] Only during exercise and upright activity

[ ] During exercise and for ___ hours after

[ ] Other: ____

2.8 When NOT to Exercise

Exercise is powerful medicine for POTS, but there are times when you should skip your session. Pushing through these situations causes crashes and setbacks.

Skip exercise if you have:

- Fever (any temperature above normal)
- Active infection (flu, COVID, significant cold, etc.)
- Severe flare of POTS symptoms beyond normal baseline
- New or worsening chest pain
- Irregular heart rhythm that feels different than usual
- Extreme fatigue that's unusual even for you
- Recent injury or acute pain

- Blood pressure significantly higher or lower than your baseline
- Severe migraine or headache
- Less than 5 hours sleep the night before

Modify or reduce exercise if you have:

- Mild cold symptoms (stuffy nose but no fever)
- Poor sleep (5-6 hours)
- Higher stress than usual
- Menstrual period (first 1-2 days—reduce intensity)
- Mild symptom flare (do half duration or lower intensity)
- Very hot weather (move to air conditioning or pool)

When in doubt, reduce the intensity or duration rather than skip completely. Consistency matters, but survival matters more. One missed session won't derail your progress. Pushing through when you shouldn't can set you back weeks.

Exercise 2.8A: Know Your Red Flags

This exercise helps you identify your personal warning signs that exercise should be modified or skipped.

Absolute "No Exercise" Signs for Me:

Check all that apply and add any personal warning signs:

[ ] Fever above _____ degrees

[ ] Active illness (specify: ____)

[ ] Heart rate above _____ while resting

[ ] Blood pressure reading above /

[ ] Blood pressure reading below /

[ ] Chest pain or unusual heart sensations

[ ] Dizziness worse than usual (rate 8+ on 1-10 scale)

[ ] Severe headache or migraine

[ ] Less than 5 hours sleep

[ ] Other personal red flag: ______________________________

[ ] Other personal red flag: ______________________________

"Modify/Reduce Exercise" Signs for Me:

[ ] Mild cold symptoms without fever

[ ] 5-6 hours of sleep

[ ] Period (first 2 days)

[ ] Stress level above _____ (on 1-10 scale)

[ ] Symptoms rated _____ or higher on personal scale

[ ] Temperature outside above _____ degrees

[ ] Other: ______________________________

When I see a red flag, I will:

____

____

____

2.9 Chapter at a Glance

- Get medical clearance from your doctor before starting any exercise program
- Establish baseline measurements for lying and standing heart rate and blood pressure
- Calculate your personal heart rate zones or plan to use RPE if on beta blockers
- Obtain essential equipment, minimally a recumbent cardio option and resistance bands
- Plan your daily sodium intake (10-12 grams) and hydration (2-3 liters)
- Consider compression garments, especially 20-30 mmHg for exercise
- Know when to skip or modify exercise to prevent setbacks
- Preparation before Day 1 determines your success throughout the program

Chapter 3.0: How to Use This Workbook

You have the knowledge. You have medical clearance. You have your equipment. Now you need to understand how this workbook actually works, day to day, week to week. This chapter is your operating manual for the next 16 weeks. Read it carefully. Return to it when you're confused. Everything you need to know about tracking, modifying, and succeeding is right here.

3.1 Program Structure Overview

This workbook is organized into 16 weeks, divided into 4 phases. Each phase has a specific purpose in your reconditioning.

Phase 1 (Weeks 1-4): Foundation

- All exercise recumbent or lying down
- Duration: 3-20 minutes per session
- Frequency: 5-6 days per week
- Intensity: Recovery to Base Pace zones
- Goal: Establish exercise habit without triggering symptoms

Phase 2 (Weeks 5-8): Building Endurance

- Continue recumbent exercise
- Duration: 20-30 minutes per session
- Frequency: 5-6 days per week
- Intensity: Base Pace to Maximal Steady State
- Goal: Increase cardiovascular capacity while still horizontal

Phase 3 (Weeks 9-12): Transition to Upright

- Begin introducing upright exercise in Week 10-11
- Duration: 25-35 minutes per session
- Frequency: 5-6 days per week
- Intensity: Variable, building tolerance to standing
- Goal: Shift from recumbent to upright exercise safely

Phase 4 (Weeks 13-16): Upright Mastery

- Primarily upright exercise
- Duration: 30-45 minutes per session

- Frequency: 5-6 days per week
- Intensity: Full range including intervals
- Goal: Establish sustainable upright exercise routine

Each week provides specific daily workouts. You'll know exactly what to do each day: which exercises, how long, what intensity, what heart rate zone. Follow the plan as written unless you need to modify for symptoms.

Exercise 3.1A: Understand the Phases

This exercise ensures you understand what happens when.

Fill in the key information for each phase:

Phase 1 (Weeks 1-4):

Position for exercise: ____

Duration range:

____

My goal for this phase: ____

____

Phase 2 (Weeks 5-8):

Position for exercise: ____

Duration range:

____

My goal for this phase: ____

____

Phase 3 (Weeks 9-12):

What changes in this phase: ____

Duration range:

____

My goal for this phase: ____

____

Phase 4 (Weeks 13-16):

Position for exercise: ____

Duration range:

____

My goal for this phase: ____

____

Which phase do I think will be hardest for me? Why?

____

____

____

3.2 Daily Tracking System

Every workout has a tracking section. You'll record specific information each time you exercise. This data shows your progress and helps identify patterns.

What to track daily:

- Date and time of exercise
- Exercise mode (recumbent bike, rowing, swimming, etc.)
- Duration (actual minutes completed)
- Heart rate zones or RPE
- How you felt during exercise (1-10 scale)
- Symptoms during exercise (if any)
- How you felt 2-4 hours after (1-10 scale)
- How you felt the next day (1-10 scale)

This seems like a lot. It's essential. You'll forget what happened last week. You'll wonder if you're improving. Your tracking log will show you the truth.

When your heart rate is 10 beats lower at Week 8 than Week 2 for the same exercise, you'll see it in your data. When you can do 25 minutes easily when 10 minutes felt hard at Week 3, you'll see it in your log. When you can stand for 15 minutes without symptoms when you could only manage 5 minutes at baseline, you'll see it.

Track everything. Every session. Use the provided templates in each week's section. This is how you prove to yourself that this is working, especially during the hard early weeks when you can't feel the changes yet.

Exercise 3.2A: Practice Tracking

This exercise helps you learn the tracking system before you start.

Complete a practice tracking log for a recent activity (like walking to your car, doing dishes, etc.):

Date: ____________________ **Time:** ____________________

Activity: ____

Duration: ____________________ **Position:** __________________________________

Heart rate during (if you measured): _________ bpm **or RPE:** _________

How I felt during (1-10, where 1=terrible, 10=great): _________

Symptoms I experienced:

____

____

How I felt 2-4 hours after (1-10): _________

How I felt the next day (1-10): _________

What this practice teaches me about tracking:

____

____

____

3.3 Modifying for Bad Days

You will have bad days. POTS is unpredictable. Your period might hit. You might get a cold. You might sleep terribly. The weather might be brutally hot. You might just wake up feeling worse than usual.

Bad days don't mean you skip completely (unless you hit a true red flag from Chapter 2.0). Bad days mean you modify intelligently.

Modification strategies:

Strategy 1 - Reduce Duration: Cut the prescribed time in half. If the workout says 20 minutes, do 10 minutes.

Strategy 2 - Lower Intensity: Drop down one zone. If prescribed Base Pace, do Recovery zone instead.

Strategy 3 - Reduce Frequency: Take an extra rest day. Come back when you feel better.

Strategy 4 - Change Mode: If upright exercise is prescribed but you feel terrible, drop back to recumbent for that day.

Strategy 5 - Just Move: Do 5 minutes of gentle movement in whatever position feels tolerable. Showing up counts.

The goal is consistency over perfection. One modified workout is infinitely better than skipping completely and losing momentum. The people who succeed are the ones who adapt to their bodies while still showing up.

Exercise 3.3A: Plan Your Modifications

This exercise helps you decide in advance how you'll modify on difficult days.

My bad day triggers: (Check all that apply)

[ ] Poor sleep (less than _____ hours)

[ ] Period (Days ___ to ___ of my cycle)

[ ] High stress

[ ] Hot weather (above _____ degrees)

[ ] POTS flare (symptoms rated _____ or higher)

[ ] Didn't get enough sodium or fluids yesterday

[ ] Other: ____

For each trigger, my modification plan:

Poor Sleep:

I will: [ ] Reduce duration by half [ ] Lower intensity one zone [ ] Take rest day [ ] Other:

____

Period:

I will: [ ] Reduce duration by half [ ] Lower intensity one zone [ ] Take rest day [ ] Other:

____

High Stress:

I will: [ ] Reduce duration by half [ ] Lower intensity one zone [ ] Take rest day [ ] Other:

____

Hot Weather:

I will: [ ] Exercise in air conditioning [ ] Switch to pool [ ] Exercise early morning [ ] Reduce intensity

POTS Flare:

I will: [ ] Reduce duration to 5-10 minutes [ ] Drop to recumbent even if upright prescribed [ ] Rest day

My rule for knowing when to modify versus rest completely:

____

____

____

3.4 Equipment Substitution Chart

You won't always have access to your primary equipment. The gym might be closed. Your recumbent bike might break. You might be traveling. This chart gives you equivalent alternatives.

Primary Equipment → Substitutes:

Recumbent Bike → Supine pedaler in bed, swimming, rowing machine, supine cycling with legs in air

Rowing Machine → Recumbent bike, resistance band rows while seated, swimming

Swimming → Recumbent bike, supine pedaler, rowing machine, any recumbent cardio

Upright Bike → Elliptical with light resistance, treadmill walking, stair stepper

Treadmill → Upright bike, elliptical, outdoor walking on flat surface

Resistance Bands → Light dumbbells, bodyweight exercises, resistance machines at gym

The key: match the position and intensity, not the exact movement. If prescribed recumbent cardio, any recumbent option works. If prescribed upright cardio, any standing cardio works. Don't let equipment be an excuse.

Exercise 3.4A: Create Your Substitution Plan

This exercise ensures you have backup options for every prescribed exercise.

My primary cardio equipment:

____

If that's unavailable, I'll substitute:

Option 1:

____

Option 2:

____

Option 3:

____

My primary strength equipment: ____

If that's unavailable, I'll substitute:

Option 1:

____

Option 2:

____

If I'm traveling, I can do:

Cardio:

____

Strength:

____

If the gym is closed or inaccessible, I can do:

Cardio:

____

Strength:

____

Equipment I absolutely cannot work around (if any):

____

My plan if I truly can't access ANY equipment:

____

____

____

3.5 Working with Hypermobility

Many POTS patients also have Ehlers-Danlos Syndrome (EDS) or Hypermobility Spectrum Disorders (HSD). If you have hypermobile joints, you need to protect them during exercise.

Key principles for hypermobility:

Never lock out joints: Keep a micro-bend in knees and elbows. Don't hyperextend.

Focus on stability over flexibility: You already have too much flexibility. Build strength that stabilizes joints.

Avoid high-impact: No jumping, no running on hard surfaces. Stick to low-impact cardio.

Use modifications: When doing strength exercises, reduce range of motion if joints feel unstable.

Support vulnerable joints: Braces for ankles, wrists, or knees if you sublux easily.

Slower is better: Control the movement through the entire range. Don't rely on momentum.

All exercises in this workbook can be modified for hypermobility. If you feel a joint becoming unstable during an exercise, stop. Reduce range of motion. Add support. Hypermobility is not a reason to skip exercise—it's a reason to exercise smarter.

Exercise 3.5A: Identify Your Needs

This exercise helps you plan for hypermobility considerations.

Do I have diagnosed EDS or HSD? [ ] Yes [ ] No [ ] Not sure

Joints that sublux or dislocate easily:

[ ] Shoulders

[ ] Elbows

[ ] Wrists

[ ] Hips

[ ] Knees

[ ] Ankles

[ ] Other: ____

For each affected joint, my protection plan:

Joint: ____________________ Protection: (Brace? Reduced range? Slower movement?)

Joint: ______________________ Protection: ____

Joint: ______________________ Protection: ____

Exercises I need to be especially careful with:

Signs a joint is becoming unstable during exercise:

What I'll do if I notice instability during a workout:

3.6 Managing MCAS Triggers

Some POTS patients also have Mast Cell Activation Syndrome (MCAS). Exercise can trigger mast cell degranulation in susceptible people, causing flushing, hives, difficulty breathing, or other allergic-type reactions.

MCAS exercise considerations:

Temperature matters: Avoid overheating. Exercise in cool environment. Use fan. Swimming in cool water is often tolerated better.

Start antihistamines before exercise: If your doctor recommends, take H1 and H2 blockers before exercising.

Watch for triggers: Heat, exertion, sweating, certain equipment materials, cleaning products on gym equipment. Identify what sets you off.

Stop if reacting: If you develop hives, flushing, wheezing, or other MCAS symptoms during exercise, stop immediately. Take prescribed rescue medication.

Keep epinephrine accessible: If you have an epi-pen prescribed for MCAS, keep it nearby during exercise.

Cool down gradually: Sudden temperature changes can trigger reactions. Cool down slowly.

Not everyone with POTS has MCAS. If you don't react to exercise with allergic-type symptoms, you can skip these precautions. If you do react, these strategies can make exercise possible.

Exercise 3.6A: MCAS Exercise Planning

This exercise helps you identify and manage MCAS triggers during exercise.

Do I have MCAS or suspected MCAS? [ ] Yes [ ] No

My typical MCAS symptoms:

[ ] Flushing/redness

[ ] Hives or rash

[ ] Itching

[ ] Difficulty breathing/wheezing

[ ] Throat tightness

[ ] Nausea or abdominal pain

[ ] Rapid heart rate (separate from POTS)

[ ] Dizziness (separate from POTS)

[ ] Other: ____

Known exercise-related triggers:

[ ] Overheating/hot environment

[ ] Sweating

[ ] Exertion level too high

[ ] Certain equipment or materials

[ ] Specific times of day

[ ] Menstrual cycle phase

[ ] Other: ____

My MCAS prevention plan for exercise:

Antihistamines I'll take before exercise: ______________________________

When I'll take them: ____

Temperature control strategies: ___________________________________

____

Emergency medications I'll keep nearby:

____

____

If I start reacting during exercise, I will:

1. ____
2. ____
3. ____

My doctor's specific instructions about exercise with MCAS:

____

____

____

3.7 Your Week by Week Plan

Starting with Week 1, each week has its own section in this workbook. Every week includes:

- Weekly goals and focus
- Daily workout prescriptions (exactly what to do each day)
- Daily tracking logs
- Weekly reflection questions
- Progress assessment

You'll work through one week at a time. Complete all prescribed workouts. Fill in all tracking logs. Answer the reflection questions. Then move to the next week.

Don't skip ahead. Don't try to speed up the progression. The timeline exists for a reason—your body needs this amount of time to adapt. Trust the process.

By Week 16, you'll look back at Week 1 and barely recognize that person. You'll be doing exercises that seemed impossible. You'll be standing and moving in ways you forgot were possible. But you have to do every week to get there.

Exercise 3.7A: Set Your Expectations

This exercise helps you commit to the week by week process.

I will complete this workbook: [ ] One week at a time [ ] I'm tempted to skip ahead (be honest)

If I'm tempted to skip ahead, I'll remember:

____

____

My plan for staying on track each week:

____

____

____

Who will hold me accountable for completing each week?

Name:

____

How they'll help:

____

____

What I'll do on my scheduled start day (Date: _______________):

____

____

____

3.8 Key Takeaways

- The program has 4 phases over 16 weeks, progressing from recumbent to upright exercise
- Track every workout using the daily logs to monitor progress and identify patterns
- Modify workouts on bad days rather than skipping completely
- Equipment substitutions are acceptable as long as position and intensity match
- Hypermobility requires joint protection: never lock out, focus on stability, use supports
- MCAS requires temperature control, antihistamines, and awareness of triggers
- Work through one week at a time without skipping ahead
- The tracking data will prove you're improving even when you can't feel it yet

PART 2: THE 16-WEEK PROGRAM

PHASE 1: FOUNDATION

(Weeks 1-4)

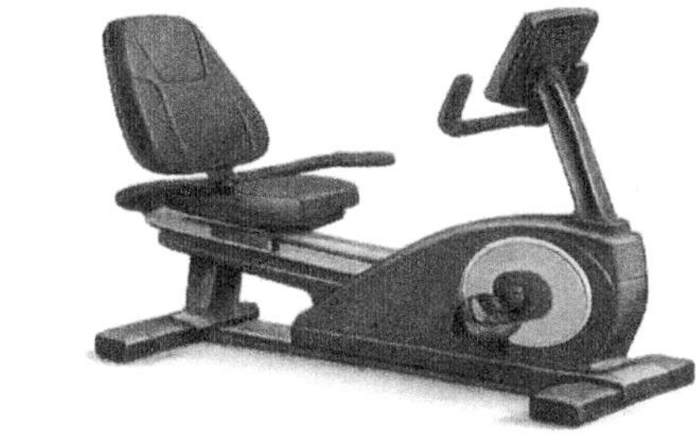

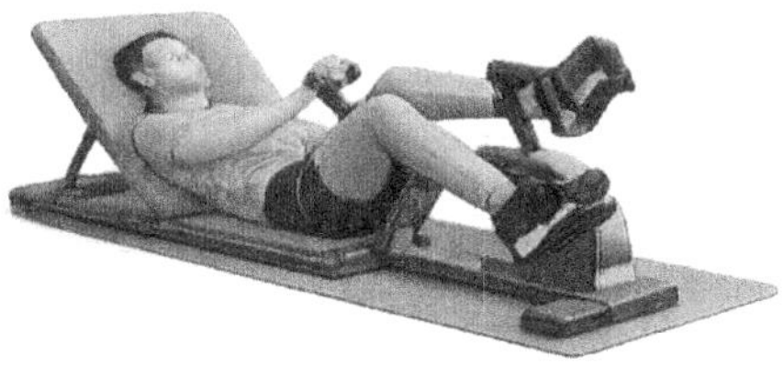

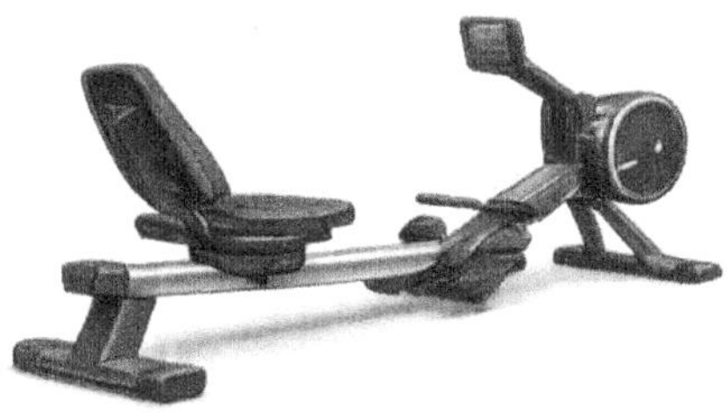

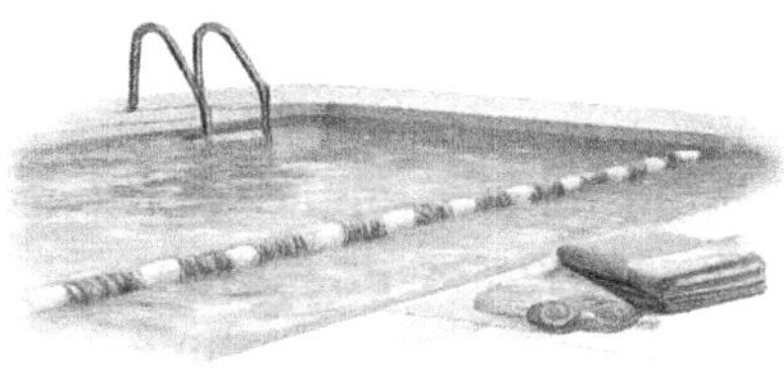

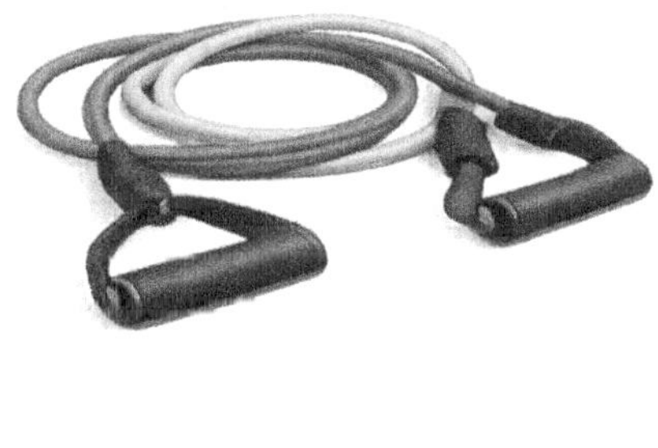

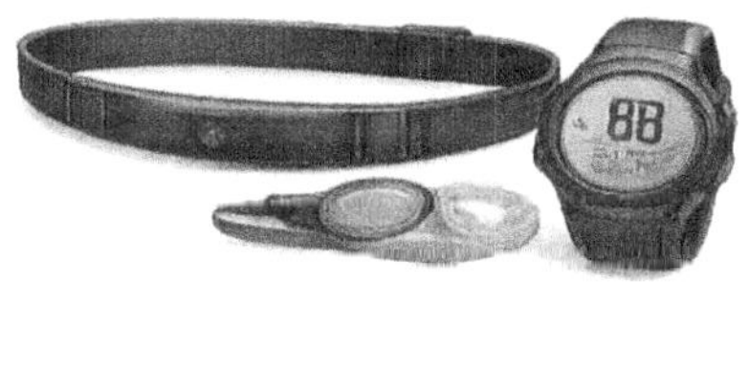

Starting Horizontal

Welcome to the foundation phase. These first four weeks establish everything. You'll start with just 3-5 minutes of recumbent exercise and build to 15-20 minutes by Week 4. You'll stay completely horizontal or recumbent—no upright exercise yet. Your body needs to learn that movement is safe before you ask it to fight gravity. Every session stays in Recovery to Base Pace zones (50-60% max heart rate). This feels easy. That's the point.

Week 1

This is it. Your first week. You're starting something that will change your body in measurable ways. This week is about establishing the habit and proving to yourself that you can exercise without crashing. You'll start with just 3-5 minutes of recumbent exercise, done 5-6 days this week. It seems almost too easy. That's intentional. You're teaching your body that movement is safe.

Week 1 Overview

Your goals this week:

- Complete 5-6 sessions of recumbent cardio (3-5 minutes each)
- Stay in Recovery Zone (50-60% max heart rate or RPE 3-4)
- Complete 2 strength training sessions (lower body and core focus)
- Track every session without fail
- Finish the week without crashing

What you'll feel: You might feel surprisingly good during exercise since you're staying horizontal and brief. Some people feel energized. Some feel cautiously optimistic. Some feel skeptical this could possibly work. All normal. By midweek, you might feel increased fatigue. Also normal. Your body is waking up.

Equipment needed: Recumbent bike, supine pedaler, rowing machine, or pool access. Resistance bands for strength training. Heart rate monitor or ability to check pulse.

If you only have 10 minutes today: Do your 3-5 minutes of cardio. That's it. The rest can wait. Consistency beats perfection.

Daily Workout Schedule

Day 1: Monday

Cardio Session:

- Equipment: Recumbent bike (or supine pedaler, rowing machine, swimming)

- Duration: 3 minutes continuous
- Intensity: Recovery Zone (50-60% max HR or RPE 3-4)
- Position: Recumbent/lying down
- Instructions: Set up your equipment. Start moving slowly. Focus on smooth, consistent motion. Check your heart rate at 1 minute and 2 minutes. Stay in your Recovery Zone. If your heart rate goes above zone, slow down immediately. Complete the full 3 minutes even if it feels easy.

Alternative if no equipment: Supine leg cycling while lying on floor or in bed. Lie on your back, lift legs, make cycling motions in the air for 3 minutes.

Day 2: Tuesday

Cardio Session:

- Equipment: Recumbent bike (or alternate)
- Duration: 3 minutes continuous
- Intensity: Recovery Zone (50-60% max HR or RPE 3-4)
- Position: Recumbent/lying down
- Instructions: Same as Day 1. Your body might feel slightly more tired today. That's expected. Still complete the full 3 minutes.

Strength Training Session 1 (after cardio or later in day):

- Leg and core exercises, all done lying or seated
- Complete the routine below
- Duration: 10-15 minutes total

Day 3: Wednesday

Cardio Session:

- Equipment: Recumbent bike (or alternate)
- Duration: 4 minutes continuous
- Intensity: Recovery Zone (50-60% max HR or RPE 3-4)
- Position: Recumbent/lying down
- Instructions: You're adding one minute. This might feel harder midway through. Check your heart rate at 2 minutes. Adjust speed if needed to stay in zone. Finish strong.

Day 4: Thursday

Cardio Session:

- Equipment: Recumbent bike (or alternate)
- Duration: 4 minutes continuous
- Intensity: Recovery Zone (50-60% max HR or RPE 3-4)
- Position: Recumbent/lying down
- Instructions: Second day at 4 minutes. Should feel slightly easier than yesterday. Your body is adapting already.

Strength Training Session 2 (after cardio or later in day):

- Leg and core exercises
- Same routine as Day 2
- Duration: 10-15 minutes total

Day 5: Friday

Cardio Session:

- Equipment: Recumbent bike (or alternate)
- Duration: 5 minutes continuous
- Intensity: Recovery Zone (50-60% max HR or RPE 3-4)
- Position: Recumbent/lying down
- Instructions: Longest session yet. Break it into mental chunks: first 2 minutes, middle minute, final 2 minutes. Check heart rate at 2.5 minutes. Stay consistent.

Day 6: Saturday

Cardio Session:

- Equipment: Recumbent bike (or alternate)
- Duration: 5 minutes continuous
- Intensity: Recovery Zone (50-60% max HR or RPE 3-4)
- Position: Recumbent/lying down
- Instructions: Final cardio session of Week 1. You've done this five times already. You know what to do.

Day 7: Sunday

Rest Day: No exercise. This is recovery. Your body needs this to adapt and grow stronger. Stay hydrated. Get extra salt. Move gently if you want but no structured exercise.

Exercise Form Guide

Recumbent Bike Form: Adjust seat so legs have slight bend at bottom of pedal stroke. Never lock knees. Sit back fully in seat. Keep shoulders relaxed. Hands rest lightly on handles. Start pedaling slowly. Build to comfortable pace. Resistance should be light enough that you can maintain steady motion for full duration. If breathing becomes labored, reduce resistance or speed.

Supine Pedaler Form: Lie flat on floor or in bed. Place pedaler near end of bed or where feet can reach comfortably. Feet go in pedal straps. Push and pull in cycling motion. Keep lower back pressed to surface. If lower back arches, bend knees slightly more. Smooth, circular motion.

Rowing Machine (Recumbent Position): Sit in seat with feet strapped in. Lean back slightly. Legs do most of work. Pull handle to lower chest. Push with legs as you pull with arms. Return slowly. Stay smooth. Don't jerk. This works whole body so monitor heart rate closely.

Swimming: Swim laps slowly, any stroke you can sustain. Rest at wall as needed. Don't race. This is about continuous gentle movement. Water keeps you cool and supports your body. Excellent option for those with joint issues.

Strength Training Routine

Complete this routine twice this week (Days 2 and 4). All exercises done lying down or seated. Do exercises in order listed. Rest 30-60 seconds between exercises. Total time: 10-15 minutes.

Supine Leg Marches (lying on back)

- Lie flat, arms at sides
- Lift one knee toward chest, lower it
- Lift other knee, lower it
- Continue alternating slowly
- Repetitions: 10 each leg (20 total)
- What it works: Hip flexors, core stability

Resistance Band Knee Extensions (seated or lying)

- Loop band around ankle and secure other end
- Straighten leg against resistance
- Slowly bend knee back
- Complete one side, then other
- Repetitions: 8-10 each leg
- What it works: Quadriceps

Glute Bridges (lying on back)

- Lie flat, knees bent, feet flat on surface
- Lift hips until body forms straight line from shoulders to knees
- Hold 2 seconds at top
- Lower slowly
- Repetitions: 8-10
- What it works: Glutes, hamstrings, core

Dead Bugs (lying on back)

- Lie flat, arms straight up toward ceiling
- Knees bent at 90 degrees, shins parallel to ground
- Lower one arm overhead while extending opposite leg
- Return to start
- Switch sides
- Repetitions: 6-8 each side
- What it works: Deep core muscles, coordination

Calf Pumps (lying or seated)

- Point toes down (like pressing gas pedal)
- Flex toes up (like pulling gas pedal back)
- Move through full range
- Can use resistance band around foot for more challenge
- Repetitions: 15-20
- What it works: Calf muscles (critical for blood return to heart)

Daily Tracking Logs

Complete one tracking log after each cardio session. This data is critical for seeing your progress.

Day 1: Date ____________

Equipment used: ____

Planned duration: __________ Actual duration completed: __________

Heart rate at start: _____ Heart rate at minute 2: _____ Heart rate at end: _____

RPE during exercise (1-10): _____

How I felt during exercise (1-10, where 10=felt great): _____

Symptoms during exercise (check all that apply): [ ] None [ ] Dizziness [ ] Nausea [ ] Heart racing beyond zone [ ] Fatigue [ ] Chest discomfort [ ] Other:
____

How I felt 2-4 hours after exercise (1-10): _____

How I felt the next morning (1-10): _____

Notes:
____

____

____

Day 2: Date ____________

Equipment used:
____

Planned duration: __________ Actual duration completed: __________

Heart rate at start: _____ Heart rate at minute 2: _____ Heart rate at end: _____

RPE during exercise (1-10): _____

How I felt during exercise (1-10): _____

Symptoms during exercise: [ ] None [ ] Dizziness [ ] Nausea [ ] Heart racing [ ] Fatigue [ ] Chest discomfort [ ] Other: ____

How I felt 2-4 hours after: _____

How I felt next morning: _____

Strength training completed: [ ] Yes [ ] No

Notes:
____

____

____

Day 3: Date ____________

Equipment used:

____

Planned duration: __________ Actual duration completed: __________

Heart rate at start: _____ Heart rate at minute 2: _____ Heart rate at end: _____

RPE during exercise (1-10): _____

How I felt during exercise (1-10): _____

Symptoms during exercise: [ ] None [ ] Dizziness [ ] Nausea [ ] Heart racing [ ] Fatigue [ ] Chest discomfort [ ] Other: ____

How I felt 2-4 hours after: _____

How I felt next morning: _____

Notes:

____

____

____

Day 4: Date ____________

Equipment used:

____

Planned duration: __________ Actual duration completed: __________

Heart rate at start: _____ Heart rate at minute 2: _____ Heart rate at end: _____

RPE during exercise (1-10): _____

How I felt during exercise (1-10): _____

Symptoms during exercise: [ ] None [ ] Dizziness [ ] Nausea [ ] Heart racing [ ] Fatigue [ ] Chest discomfort [ ] Other: ____

How I felt 2-4 hours after: _____

How I felt next morning: _____

Strength training completed: [ ] Yes [ ] No

Notes:

____

____

____

Day 5: Date _____________

Equipment used:

____

Planned duration: __________ Actual duration completed: __________

Heart rate at start: _____ Heart rate at minute 2: _____ Heart rate at end: _____

RPE during exercise (1-10): _____

How I felt during exercise (1-10): _____

Symptoms during exercise: [ ] None [ ] Dizziness [ ] Nausea [ ] Heart racing [ ] Fatigue [ ] Chest discomfort [ ] Other: ____

How I felt 2-4 hours after: _____

How I felt next morning: _____

Notes:

____

____

____

Day 6: Date _____________

Equipment used:

____

Planned duration: __________ Actual duration completed: __________

Heart rate at start: _____ Heart rate at minute 2: _____ Heart rate at end: _____

RPE during exercise (1-10): _____

How I felt during exercise (1-10): _____

Symptoms during exercise: [ ] None [ ] Dizziness [ ] Nausea [ ] Heart racing [ ] Fatigue [ ] Chest discomfort [ ] Other: ____

How I felt 2-4 hours after: _____

How I felt next morning: _____

Notes:

____

____

____

Recovery Strategies

Recovery is when your body actually gets stronger. Exercise breaks down tissue. Recovery builds it back stronger. This week, prioritize these recovery strategies:

Hydration: Drink 2-3 liters of fluid daily. More on exercise days. Front-load fluids before exercise. Drink 8-16 oz with electrolytes 30-60 minutes before each session.

Salt loading: Continue your daily sodium target (10-12 grams). Take extra salt 30 minutes before exercise if your doctor approves.

Sleep: Aim for 8-9 hours. POTS patients need more sleep than typical people. Set consistent bedtime. Keep room cool. Elevate head of bed 4-6 inches.

Compression: Wear compression garments during all upright activity and exercise. Put them on before standing in morning. Keep them on until you're lying down for extended periods.

Post-exercise protocol: After each session, stay horizontal for 15-30 minutes. Drink 16-24 oz of fluid with sodium. Don't jump up immediately. Let your system settle.

Gentle movement: On rest days, gentle movement is fine. Walking slowly, gentle stretching, easy yoga. Nothing that elevates heart rate or causes symptoms.

My Recovery Plan:

Daily hydration goal: __________ liters

Daily sodium goal: __________ grams

Sleep goal: __________ hours per night (Bedtime: ________ Wake: ________)

Post-exercise routine I'll follow:

____

____

____

What If I Crash

If you crash this week despite following the protocol, here's what to do.

First, identify if it's actually a crash or expected fatigue. Crash means: symptoms significantly worse than baseline for 24+ hours, unable to do normal activities, feel like you're back to square one. Expected fatigue means: more tired than usual, slight increase in symptoms, but can still function.

If it's expected fatigue (most likely):

- Take an extra rest day
- Drop next session to 3 minutes instead of prescribed duration
- Lower intensity to very easy (RPE 2-3)
- Keep showing up but back off temporarily
- This will pass in a few days

If it's a true crash:

- Take 2-3 days complete rest
- When you restart, go back to Day 1 prescription (3 minutes)
- Stay there until you can complete it without increased symptoms

- Then progress by adding 1 minute every 3-4 days
- Figure out what triggered it: Did you go too hard? Not enough hydration? Illness brewing? Inadequate sleep?

Most common crash triggers Week 1:

- Going above prescribed heart rate zone
- Exercising when already having a POTS flare
- Inadequate hydration or sodium
- Poor sleep night before
- Fighting off an infection
- Doing exercise in upright position instead of recumbent

My early warning signs that I might crash:

Physical signs:

____

____

Symptom changes:

____

____

If I experience expected fatigue this week, I will:

____

____

____

If I crash this week, I will:

Step 1:

____

Step 2:

____

Step 3:

____

Week 1 Reflection

Complete this at the end of Day 7. Look back at your tracking logs.

Sessions completed this week: _____ out of 6 planned cardio sessions

Strength sessions completed: _____ out of 2 planned

Total minutes of cardio this week: _____ minutes

What went well:

What was harder than expected:

Biggest surprise this week:

How my body felt by end of week compared to beginning:

One thing I'll do differently in Week 2:

Rate my confidence level going into Week 2 (1-10): _____

Why I rated it that way:

Week 2

You did Week 1. You showed up. You didn't crash. Your body is starting to remember what exercise feels like. This week builds on that foundation. You'll increase duration to 5-8 minutes per session and add slight variety to your cardio. Everything stays recumbent. You're still proving to your body that movement is safe and tolerable.

Week 2 Overview

Your goals this week:

- Complete 5-6 sessions of recumbent cardio (5-8 minutes each)
- Continue Recovery to low Base Pace Zone (50-65% max heart rate or RPE 3-5)
- Complete 2 strength training sessions (progressing from Week 1)
- Try at least one different equipment type if available
- Track patterns between exercise and symptoms
- Build on Week 1 without increasing fatigue

What you'll feel: This week often feels harder than Week 1, not because the exercise is that much longer, but because cumulative fatigue builds. This is normal. Your body is adapting. You might feel more tired midweek. You might sleep longer. You might need more rest periods during the day. All expected. By weekend, you might start feeling slightly stronger during exercise.

Equipment needed: Same as Week 1. If possible, try a different piece of equipment for at least one session this week to add variety.

Weekly challenge: Complete all 6 cardio sessions without skipping. Consistency matters more than perfection.

Daily Workout Schedule

Day 1: Monday

- Equipment: Recumbent bike
- Duration: 5 minutes continuous
- Intensity: Recovery Zone (50-60% max HR or RPE 3-4)
- Instructions: Starting where you left off last week. Five minutes should feel manageable after doing it twice in Week 1.

Day 2: Tuesday

- Equipment: Rowing machine (or recumbent bike if no rowing access)
- Duration: 6 minutes continuous
- Intensity: Recovery to low Base Pace (55-65% max HR or RPE 4-5)
- Instructions: Adding one minute and trying different equipment if possible. Rowing engages more muscle groups so monitor heart rate closely.
- Strength Training Session 1 (increased reps from Week 1)

Day 3: Wednesday

- Equipment: Recumbent bike
- Duration: 6 minutes continuous
- Intensity: Recovery to low Base Pace (55-65% max HR or RPE 4-5)
- Instructions: Second day at 6 minutes. Split it mentally: 3 minutes, then 3 more.

Day 4: Thursday

- Equipment: Swimming (or recumbent bike if no pool)
- Duration: 7 minutes continuous movement
- Intensity: Recovery Zone (50-60% max HR or RPE 3-4)
- Instructions: Longest session yet. If swimming, rest briefly at wall as needed but keep moving.
- Strength Training Session 2

Day 5: Friday

- Equipment: Recumbent bike
- Duration: 8 minutes continuous
- Intensity: Recovery to low Base Pace (55-65% max HR or RPE 4-5)
- Instructions: Peak duration for Week 2. Break it into 4-minute chunks mentally.

Day 6: Saturday

- Equipment: Your choice (any recumbent option)
- Duration: 8 minutes continuous
- Intensity: Recovery to low Base Pace (55-65% max HR or RPE 4-5)
- Instructions: Final session of Week 2. Choose the equipment you enjoy most.

Day 7: Sunday

- Rest Day: Complete rest. No structured exercise.

Strength Training Progression

This week's strength training builds on Week 1 by increasing repetitions and adding one new exercise.

Week 2 Strength Routine (Days 2 and 4):

Supine Leg Marches

- Repetitions: 12 each leg (24 total) - increased from 10

Resistance Band Knee Extensions

- Repetitions: 10-12 each leg - increased from 8-10

Glute Bridges

- Repetitions: 10-12 - increased from 8-10

Dead Bugs

- Repetitions: 8-10 each side - increased from 6-8

Calf Pumps

- Repetitions: 20-25 - increased from 15-20

NEW: Side-Lying Leg Lifts (added Week 2)

- Lie on side, bottom leg bent for stability
- Top leg straight, lift up toward ceiling
- Hold 1 second at top
- Lower slowly without touching bottom leg
- Complete one side, flip, do other side
- Repetitions: 8-10 each leg
- What it works: Hip stabilizers, important for upright exercise later

Daily Tracking Logs

Day 1: Date ____________

Equipment: ______________________________ Duration: _________

Start HR: _____ Mid HR: _____ End HR: _____ RPE: _____

During exercise (1-10): _____ Symptoms: ____

2-4 hours after (1-10): _____ Next morning (1-10): _____

Notes:

____

____

Day 2: Date ____________

Equipment: ______________________________ Duration: __________

Start HR: _____ Mid HR: _____ End HR: _____ RPE: _____

During exercise (1-10): _____ Symptoms: ____

2-4 hours after (1-10): _____ Next morning (1-10): _____

Strength training: [ ] Completed

Notes:

____

____

Day 3: Date ____________

Equipment: ______________________________ Duration: __________

Start HR: _____ Mid HR: _____ End HR: _____ RPE: _____

During exercise (1-10): _____ Symptoms: ____

2-4 hours after (1-10): _____ Next morning (1-10): _____

Notes:

____

____

Day 4: Date ____________

Equipment: ______________________________ Duration: _________

Start HR: _____ Mid HR: _____ End HR: _____ RPE: _____

During exercise (1-10): _____ Symptoms: _____________________________________

2-4 hours after (1-10): _____ Next morning (1-10): _____

Strength training: [ ] Completed

Notes:

____

Day 5: Date ____________

Equipment: ______________________________ Duration: _________

Start HR: _____ Mid HR: _____ End HR: _____ RPE: _____

During exercise (1-10): _____ Symptoms: _____________________________________

2-4 hours after (1-10): _____ Next morning (1-10): _____

Notes:

____

Day 6: Date ____________

Equipment: ______________________________ Duration: _________

Start HR: _____ Mid HR: _____ End HR: _____ RPE: _____

During exercise (1-10): _____ Symptoms: _____________________________________

2-4 hours after (1-10): _____ Next morning (1-10): _____

Notes:

____

Pattern Recognition

By end of Week 2, you have 12 cardio sessions tracked. That's enough data to spot patterns.

Review your tracking logs from Week 1 and Week 2. Answer these questions:

What time of day do I feel best during exercise?

Morning: Average feeling (1-10): _____

Afternoon: Average feeling (1-10): _____

Evening: Average feeling (1-10): _____

Best time for me:

____

Which equipment type do I tolerate best?

____

Days I felt best the next morning after exercise:

Dates:

____

What was similar about those days: ______________________________

____

Days I felt worse after exercise:

Dates:

____

What was different about those days: ______________________________

____

Connection between hydration and how I feel:

Days I drank 2+ liters: Feel rating: _____

Days I drank less than 2 liters: Feel rating: _____

Connection between sleep and exercise tolerance:

Days with 8+ hours sleep: Tolerance: ____

Days with less than 7 hours: Tolerance: ____

Biggest pattern I notice:

____

____

How I'll use this information in Week 3:

____

____

Managing Midweek Fatigue

Most people hit increased fatigue Wednesday or Thursday of Week 2. This is when many people question if the protocol is working. It is. Here's why you're more tired.

Your body is doing real work. Even 5-8 minutes of exercise is stimulus your deconditioned system isn't used to. Your muscles are repairing. Your cardiovascular system is adapting. This all requires energy. The fatigue is your body saying "I'm working on changes here."

What to do about midweek fatigue:

- Sleep more. Add 30-60 minutes if possible.
- Increase sodium and fluid intake.
- Take scheduled rest breaks during day, lying down 15-30 minutes.
- Simplify other activities. Don't add additional stressors this week.
- Keep doing your prescribed exercise anyway.
- Trust that this will pass. By Week 3-4, the fatigue typically decreases.

My Fatigue Management Plan:

Current fatigue level (1-10): _____

Strategies I'll use this week:

Sleep:

____

Hydration:

____

Rest breaks:

____

Activity reduction: ____

Week 2 Reflection

Sessions completed: _____ out of 6 cardio, _____ out of 2 strength

Total cardio minutes this week: _____ minutes

Total cardio minutes Week 1: _____ minutes

How Week 2 compared to Week 1:

Physical difficulty: [ ] Easier [ ] About the same [ ] Harder

Fatigue level: [ ] Less tired [ ] About the same [ ] More tired

Confidence: [ ] Higher [ ] About the same [ ] Lower

Most valuable thing I learned this week:

____

____

Biggest challenge this week:

____

____

One thing I'm proud of from this week:

____

My goal for Week 3:

Week 3

You're halfway through Phase 1. Your body has done 12 cardio sessions. You've built from 3 minutes to 8 minutes. This week pushes to 10-12 minutes per session. You're still completely recumbent. Still in Recovery to Base Pace zones. But the duration is getting real. Ten minutes of continuous exercise is significant when you started unable to tolerate any movement. Believe you can do this.

Week 3 Overview

Your goals this week:

- Complete 5-6 sessions of recumbent cardio (8-12 minutes each)
- Continue Recovery to Base Pace Zone (50-65% max heart rate or RPE 3-5)
- Complete 2 strength training sessions (further progression)
- Add one session at true Base Pace (60-70% max HR or RPE 5-6) if tolerated
- Notice improvements in how exercise feels
- Continue building without setbacks

What you'll feel: Many people report this is the week things start to click. Exercise begins feeling more doable. Recovery after sessions improves. You might notice less post-exercise fatigue. Some people feel genuinely good during exercise for the first time. Don't get cocky and jump ahead, but acknowledge this progress. Your body is changing.

Equipment needed: Same as previous weeks. Continue varying equipment to prevent boredom.

Key focus: Completing the full prescribed duration at each session. Ten to twelve minutes can feel long mentally even when your body can handle it. Break it into chunks.

Daily Workout Schedule

Day 1: Monday

- Equipment: Recumbent bike
- Duration: 8 minutes continuous
- Intensity: Recovery Zone (50-60% max HR or RPE 3-4)
- Instructions: Starting week at 8 minutes, which was your peak last week. Should feel manageable.

Day 2: Tuesday

- Equipment: Rowing machine (or alternate)
- Duration: 10 minutes continuous
- Intensity: Recovery to Base Pace (55-65% max HR or RPE 4-5)
- Instructions: Breaking into double digits. This is milestone territory. Check heart rate at 5 minutes. Adjust if needed.
- Strength Training Session 1

Day 3: Wednesday

- Equipment: Recumbent bike
- Duration: 10 minutes continuous
- Intensity: Base Pace (60-70% max HR or RPE 5-6)
- Instructions: First session at true Base Pace if you tolerated Day 2 well. You should feel like you're working but can still hold a conversation. If this feels too hard, drop back to Recovery Zone.

Day 4: Thursday

- Equipment: Swimming (or alternate)
- Duration: 12 minutes continuous
- Intensity: Recovery Zone (50-60% max HR or RPE 3-4)
- Instructions: Longest session yet. Twelve continuous minutes. Break into 3-minute chunks mentally. You can do this.
- Strength Training Session 2

Day 5: Friday

- Equipment: Recumbent bike
- Duration: 12 minutes continuous
- Intensity: Recovery to Base Pace (55-65% max HR or RPE 4-5)
- Instructions: Second day at 12 minutes. Should feel slightly easier than Day 4.

Day 6: Saturday

- Equipment: Your choice
- Duration: 12 minutes continuous
- Intensity: Base Pace (60-70% max HR or RPE 5-6)
- Instructions: Final session of Week 3. You're ending this week with 12 solid minutes at Base Pace. That's real cardiovascular work.

Day 7: Sunday

- Rest Day: Complete rest. Reflect on three weeks completed.

Strength Training Progression

Week 3 increases repetitions again and adds another new exercise.

Week 3 Strength Routine (Days 2 and 4):

Supine Leg Marches

- Repetitions: 15 each leg (30 total)

Resistance Band Knee Extensions

- Repetitions: 12-15 each leg

Glute Bridges

- Repetitions: 12-15

Dead Bugs

- Repetitions: 10-12 each side

Calf Pumps

- Repetitions: 25-30

Side-Lying Leg Lifts

- Repetitions: 10-12 each leg

NEW: Supine Hip Abduction (added Week 3)

- Lie on back, knees bent, feet flat, resistance band around thighs just above knees
- Press knees apart against band resistance
- Hold 2 seconds
- Return slowly
- Repetitions: 12-15
- What it works: Hip abductors, glutes (critical for pelvic stability during upright activity)

Daily Tracking Logs

Day 1: Date _____________

Equipment: _____________________ Duration: _____ HR Start/Mid/End: //_____

RPE: _____ During (1-10): _____ After (1-10): _____ Next AM (1-10): _____

Symptoms:

____

Notes:

____

Day 2: Date _____________

Equipment: _____________________ Duration: _____ HR Start/Mid/End: //_____

RPE: _____ During (1-10): _____ After (1-10): _____ Next AM (1-10): _____

Symptoms:

____

Strength: [ ] Completed

Notes:

____

Day 3: Date _____________

Equipment: _____________________ Duration: _____ HR Start/Mid/End: //_____

RPE: _____ During (1-10): _____ After (1-10): _____ Next AM (1-10): _____

Symptoms:

____

Notes:

____

Day 4: Date _____________

Equipment: _____________________ Duration: _____ HR Start/Mid/End: //_____

RPE: _____ During (1-10): _____ After (1-10): _____ Next AM (1-10): _____

Symptoms:

____

Strength: [ ] Completed

Notes:

____

Day 5: Date ____________

Equipment: ____________________ Duration: _____ HR Start/Mid/End: //_____

RPE: _____ During (1-10): _____ After (1-10): _____ Next AM (1-10): _____

Symptoms:

____

Notes:

____

Day 6: Date ____________

Equipment: ____________________ Duration: _____ HR Start/Mid/End: //_____

RPE: _____ During (1-10): _____ After (1-10): _____ Next AM (1-10): _____

Symptoms:

____

Notes:

____

Mental Strategies for Longer Duration

Twelve minutes can feel psychologically long even when your body can handle it. Here are strategies to manage the mental game:

Chunking: Break 12 minutes into four 3-minute segments. Count down segments instead of total time.

Distraction: Listen to music, podcast, or audiobook. Choose upbeat music with good rhythm for cardio.

Focus on form: Pay attention to technique. Smooth pedal stroke. Relaxed shoulders. Even breathing.

Heart rate checks: Use checking your heart rate as mental milestones. Check at 4 minutes, 8 minutes, and completion.

Positive self-talk: "I can do anything for 3 more minutes." "My body is getting stronger." "This is working."

Visualization: Picture your heart growing larger. Imagine your blood vessels becoming more efficient. See yourself doing activities you can't do now.

My Mental Strategy:

What I'll think about during exercise: ____

Music/audio I'll use: ____

How I'll break up the time: ____

Phrase I'll repeat when it gets hard: _______________________________________

Week 3 Reflection

Sessions completed: _____ out of 6 cardio, _____ out of 2 strength

Total cardio minutes this week: _____ minutes

Longest single session: _____ minutes

Improvements I notice from Week 1:

Physical:

____

Mental/emotional:

Symptoms:

How 10-12 minute sessions felt compared to 3-5 minute sessions:

Confidence level now (1-10): _____

What's contributing to that confidence:

Looking ahead to Week 4 (final week of Phase 1):

Week 4

Final week of Phase 1. You're going to hit 15-20 minutes per session this week. That's significant cardiovascular work for a POTS patient who couldn't exercise three weeks ago. You'll stay recumbent for these longer durations. By Saturday, you'll complete 20 continuous minutes. That's your Phase 1 graduation requirement. Finish strong.

Week 4 Overview

Your goals this week:

- Complete 5-6 sessions of recumbent cardio (15-20 minutes each)
- Work primarily in Base Pace Zone (60-70% max heart rate or RPE 5-6)
- Complete 2 strength training sessions (peak intensity for Phase 1)
- Successfully complete 20 minutes continuous on final session
- Finish Phase 1 without setbacks
- Prepare mentally for Phase 2 next week

What you'll feel: This week requires real focus. Twenty minutes is long enough that mental endurance matters as much as physical. You might feel genuinely tired during sessions. That's appropriate. You're doing actual cardiovascular work now. Post-exercise, you should feel accomplished but not destroyed. If you're crashing after sessions, you're going too hard. Drop intensity, not duration.

Equipment needed: Same as previous weeks. Choose equipment that allows you to sustain 20 minutes comfortably.

Week 4 milestone: Completing 20 continuous minutes of recumbent cardio at Base Pace is your Phase 1 completion marker. Everything you've done has built to this. You're ready.

Daily Workout Schedule

Day 1: Monday

- Equipment: Recumbent bike
- Duration: 15 minutes continuous
- Intensity: Base Pace (60-70% max HR or RPE 5-6)
- Instructions: Jumping from 12 to 15 minutes. First session at this duration. Check heart rate every 5 minutes. Stay in zone.

Day 2: Tuesday

- Equipment: Rowing machine (or alternate)
- Duration: 15 minutes continuous
- Intensity: Base Pace (60-70% max HR or RPE 5-6)
- Instructions: Second day at 15 minutes. Break into three 5-minute blocks mentally.
- Strength Training Session 1

Day 3: Wednesday

- Equipment: Recumbent bike
- Duration: 18 minutes continuous
- Intensity: Base Pace (60-70% max HR or RPE 5-6)
- Instructions: Building toward 20. Eighteen minutes requires sustained focus. You're almost there.

Day 4: Thursday

- Equipment: Swimming (or alternate)
- Duration: 18 minutes continuous
- Intensity: Recovery to Base Pace (55-65% max HR or RPE 4-5)
- Instructions: Second day at 18 minutes. Slightly lower intensity to ensure you recover for weekend push.
- Strength Training Session 2

Day 5: Friday

- Equipment: Recumbent bike
- Duration: 20 minutes continuous
- Intensity: Base Pace (60-70% max HR or RPE 5-6)
- Instructions: Twenty minutes. This is it. The duration you've been building toward. You can do this. Check heart rate at 5, 10, and 15 minutes. Stay steady.

Day 6: Saturday

- Equipment: Your choice
- Duration: 20 minutes continuous
- Intensity: Base Pace (60-70% max HR or RPE 5-6)
- Instructions: Final session of Phase 1. Twenty continuous minutes at Base Pace on your preferred equipment. This is your Phase 1 graduation session. Make it count.

Day 7: Sunday

- Rest Day: Celebrate completing Phase 1. Reflect on four weeks of progress. Prepare for Phase 2.

Strength Training Peak

Week 4 represents peak load for Phase 1 strength training. Phase 2 will introduce new exercises, so this week maximizes your current routine.

Week 4 Strength Routine (Days 2 and 4):

Supine Leg Marches

- Repetitions: 20 each leg (40 total)

Resistance Band Knee Extensions

- Repetitions: 15 each leg

Glute Bridges

- Repetitions: 15

Dead Bugs

- Repetitions: 12 each side

Calf Pumps

- Repetitions: 30

Side-Lying Leg Lifts

- Repetitions: 12-15 each leg

Supine Hip Abduction

- Repetitions: 15

Daily Tracking Logs

Day 1: Date _____________

Equipment: ______________________ Duration: _____ HR Start/Mid/End: //_____

RPE: _____ During (1-10): _____ After (1-10): _____ Next AM (1-10): _____

How 15 minutes felt:

____

Notes:

____

Day 2: Date ____________

Equipment: ____________________ Duration: _____ HR Start/Mid/End: //_____

RPE: _____ During (1-10): _____ After (1-10): _____ Next AM (1-10): _____

Strength: [ ] Completed

Notes:

____

Day 3: Date ____________

Equipment: ____________________ Duration: _____ HR Start/Mid/End: //_____

RPE: _____ During (1-10): _____ After (1-10): _____ Next AM (1-10): _____

Notes:

____

Day 4: Date ____________

Equipment: ____________________ Duration: _____ HR Start/Mid/End: //_____

RPE: _____ During (1-10): _____ After (1-10): _____ Next AM (1-10): _____

Strength: [ ] Completed

Notes:

____

Day 5: Date ____________

Equipment: ____________________ Duration: _____ HR Start/Mid/End: //_____

RPE: _____ During (1-10): _____ After (1-10): _____ Next AM (1-10): _____

How completing 20 minutes felt:

Notes:

Day 6: Date _____________

Equipment: ______________________ Duration: _____ HR Start/Mid/End: //_____

RPE: _____ During (1-10): _____ After (1-10): _____ Next AM (1-10): _____

Phase 1 completion - how I feel:

Notes:

Preparing for Phase 2

Phase 2 starts next week. Here's what changes:

- Duration increases to 20-30 minutes per session
- Intensity pushes into Maximal Steady State (70-80% max HR)
- Introduction of interval concepts
- New strength exercises focusing on core and leg power
- Everything still remains recumbent

What to expect: Phase 2 is harder. You'll be working at higher intensities for longer durations. The fatigue might return temporarily as your body adapts to new demands. This is expected. You've built the foundation. Now you're building the structure.

My readiness for Phase 2:

Do I feel ready: [ ] Yes [ ] Somewhat [ ] Not yet

If not yet, what concerns me: ____

What I've learned in Phase 1 that will help me in Phase 2:

Phase 1 Complete Assessment

Total sessions completed in Phase 1: _____ out of 24 cardio, _____ out of 8 strength

Total cardio minutes in Phase 1: _____ minutes

Week 1 total minutes: _____ **Week 4 total minutes:** _____ **Increase:** _____ minutes

Physical changes I notice:

During exercise:

After exercise:

Daily symptoms:

Standing tolerance: ______________________________

Measurements to retake:

Complete the same baseline measurements you did before Week 1. Compare the results.

Lying heart rate today: _____ **Baseline (before Week 1):** _____

Standing heart rate (1 minute): _____ Baseline: _____

Standing heart rate (3 minutes): _____ Baseline: _____

Standing tolerance time: _____ Baseline: _____

Changes in measurements:

Most significant accomplishment from Phase 1:

Biggest challenge I overcame:

What I learned about my body:

Confidence going into Phase 2 (1-10): _____

I'm ready bccause:

PHASE 2: BUILDING ENDURANCE (Weeks 5-8)

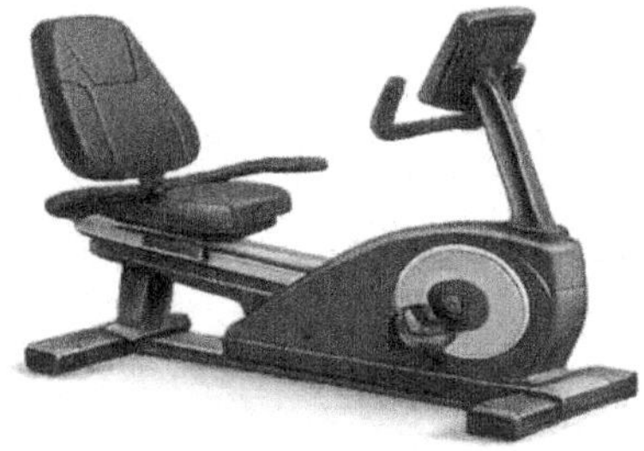
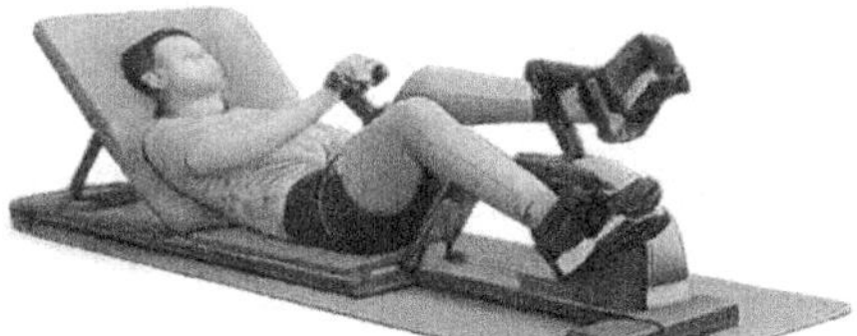
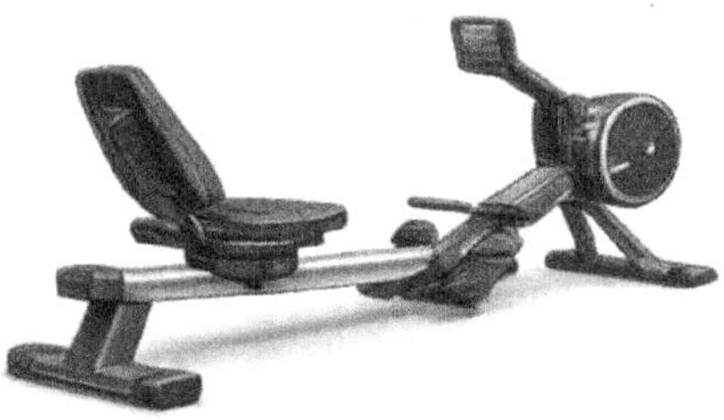
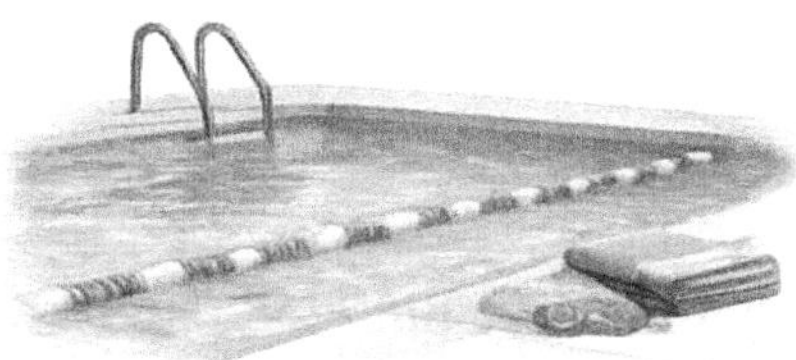
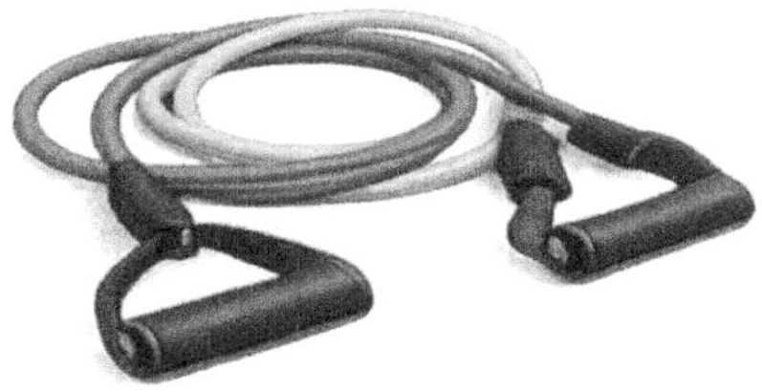
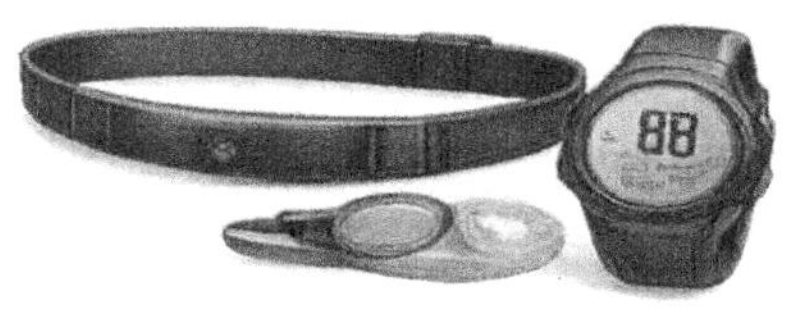

Increasing Time and Intensity

You completed Phase 1. You built from 3 minutes to 20 minutes of continuous recumbent exercise. Your heart is already larger than it was four weeks ago. Your blood volume has increased. Your muscles are stronger. Now you build on that foundation. Phase 2 increases both duration (20-30 minutes) and intensity (Base Pace to Maximal Steady State). You'll introduce interval concepts. You'll strengthen your core and legs more aggressively.

Everything still stays recumbent. You're not ready for upright yet. But you're building the cardiovascular capacity that will make upright possible in Phase 3.

Week 5

Welcome to Phase 2. This week increases both time and intensity. You'll work in the 20-25 minute range, and you'll spend more time in Base Pace Zone (60-70% max HR). You'll also get your first introduction to intervals—short bursts of slightly higher intensity followed by recovery. Your body can handle more now. Time to challenge it.

Week 5 Overview

Your goals this week:

- Complete 5-6 sessions of recumbent cardio (20-25 minutes each)
- Work primarily in Base Pace Zone (60-70% max HR or RPE 5-6)
- Include one interval introduction session
- Complete 2 strength training sessions (new exercises added)
- Maintain consistency without increased symptoms
- Trust that you can handle longer, harder work

What you'll feel: The jump to consistent 20+ minute sessions might feel like a lot initially. By midweek, your body adapts. The intervals might spike your heart rate unexpectedly. That's normal. You're teaching your body to recover quickly from increased demands. Some fatigue is expected early in Phase 2. It typically resolves by Week 6-7.

Equipment needed: Same recumbent options. Intervals work on any equipment.

Key focus: Completing full duration even when mentally challenging. Twenty-five minutes is long enough that boredom or mental fatigue can be the limiting factor, not physical capacity.

Daily Workout Schedule

Day 1: Monday

- Equipment: Recumbent bike
- Duration: 20 minutes continuous
- Intensity: Base Pace (60-70% max HR or RPE 5-6)

- Instructions: Starting Phase 2 at 20 minutes, your ending point from Phase 1. Establish baseline for this phase.

Day 2: Tuesday

- Equipment: Rowing machine (or alternate)
- Duration: 22 minutes continuous
- Intensity: Base Pace (60-70% max HR or RPE 5-6)
- Instructions: Adding 2 minutes. Check heart rate at 10 minutes and 20 minutes.
- Strength Training Session 1 (new exercises)

Day 3: Wednesday

- Equipment: Recumbent bike
- Duration: 20 minutes with intervals
- Intensity: Base Pace with brief Maximal Steady State intervals
- Instructions: **Interval Introduction**
    - Warm up 5 minutes in Recovery Zone
    - Minutes 6-15: Alternate 2 minutes Base Pace, 1 minute Maximal Steady State (70-80% max HR or RPE 6-7)
    - Complete 5 intervals total
    - Cool down 5 minutes in Recovery Zone
- This introduces your body to intensity changes. Heart rate will spike during intervals. That's expected.

Day 4: Thursday

- Equipment: Swimming (or alternate)
- Duration: 22 minutes continuous
- Intensity: Base Pace (60-70% max HR or RPE 5-6)
- Instructions: No intervals today. Steady state work to recover from yesterday.
- Strength Training Session 2

Day 5: Friday

- Equipment: Recumbent bike
- Duration: 25 minutes continuous
- Intensity: Base Pace (60-70% max HR or RPE 5-6)
- Instructions: Longest session of Week 5. Twenty-five continuous minutes. Break into five 5-minute blocks.

Day 6: Saturday

- Equipment: Your choice
- Duration: 25 minutes continuous
- Intensity: Base Pace to Maximal Steady State (65-75% max HR or RPE 5-7)
- Instructions: Final session of Week 5. You're ending this week with 25 solid minutes at higher average intensity.

Day 7: Sunday

- Rest Day

Understanding Intervals

Intervals are short periods of higher intensity followed by recovery periods. They teach your body to:

- Recover quickly from increased demands
- Work at higher intensities briefly
- Build cardiovascular capacity faster than steady state alone
- Prepare for the variability of real life (walking up stairs, carrying groceries, etc.)

Interval structure this week:

- Work interval: 1 minute at Maximal Steady State (70-80% max HR)
- Recovery interval: 2 minutes at Base Pace
- You're alternating between working harder and backing off
- Total work time is short (5 minutes total at higher intensity out of 20-minute session)

If intervals spike your heart rate too high:

- Reduce the work interval to 30 seconds instead of 1 minute
- Keep recovery intervals at 2 minutes
- It's fine if heart rate goes to 75-80% max HR during work intervals
- What matters is that it comes back down during recovery

New Strength Exercises

Phase 2 adds exercises that build power and core stability needed for eventual upright exercise.

Week 5 Strength Routine (Days 2 and 4):

Continue from Phase 1:

- Supine Leg Marches: 20 each leg
- Resistance Band Knee Extensions: 15 each leg
- Glute Bridges: 15
- Dead Bugs: 12 each side
- Calf Pumps: 30
- Side-Lying Leg Lifts: 15 each leg
- Supine Hip Abduction: 15

NEW: Single-Leg Glute Bridge

- Lie on back, one foot flat, other leg extended straight
- Lift hips using single leg
- Hold 2 seconds
- Lower slowly
- Complete all reps one side, then switch
- Repetitions: 6-8 each leg
- What it works: Unilateral glute and hamstring strength

NEW: Supine Bicycle Crunches

- Lie on back, hands behind head lightly
- Lift shoulders slightly off ground
- Bring opposite elbow toward opposite knee while extending other leg
- Alternate sides in cycling motion
- Repetitions: 20 total (10 each side)
- What it works: Obliques, deep core, coordination

Daily Tracking Logs

Day 1: Date _____________

Equipment: ______________________ Duration: _____ HR Start/Mid/End: //_____

RPE: _____ During (1-10): _____ After (1-10): _____ Next AM (1-10): _____

Notes:

____

Day 2: Date _____________

Equipment: ______________________ Duration: _____ HR Start/Mid/End: //_____

RPE: _____ During (1-10): _____ After (1-10): _____ Next AM (1-10): _____

Strength: [ ] Completed

Notes:

____

Day 3: Date _____________ (Interval Day)

Equipment: _____________________ Duration: _____

Warm-up HR: _____ Peak interval HR: _____ Recovery HR after intervals: _____

RPE during intervals: _____ During (1-10): _____ After (1-10): _____ Next AM (1-10): _____

How intervals felt:

____

____

Notes:

____

Day 4: Date _____________

Equipment: _____________________ Duration: _____ HR Start/Mid/End: //_____

RPE: _____ During (1-10): _____ After (1-10): _____ Next AM (1-10): _____

Strength: [ ] Completed

Notes:

____

Day 5: Date _____________

Equipment: _____________________ Duration: _____ HR Start/Mid/End: //_____

RPE: _____ During (1-10): _____ After (1-10): _____ Next AM (1-10): _____

How 25 minutes felt:

____

Notes:

____

Day 6: Date _____________

Equipment: ______________________ Duration: _____ HR Start/Mid/End: //_____

RPE: _____ During (1-10): _____ After (1-10): _____ Next AM (1-10): _____

Notes:

____

Week 5 Reflection

Sessions completed: _____ out of 6 cardio, _____ out of 2 strength

Total cardio minutes this week: _____ minutes

How intervals felt:

____

____

How 25-minute sessions felt compared to 20-minute sessions:

____

____

Energy level this week compared to Week 4:

[ ] More energetic [ ] About the same [ ] More fatigued

Adjustments I need to make for Week 6:

____

____

Confidence level (1-10): _____

Week 6

You survived your first week of Phase 2 and introduction to intervals. This week continues building: 25-30 minutes per session, more time in Maximal Steady State zone, and expanded interval work. Your body is adapting to higher demands. Trust that you can handle this.

Week 6 Overview

Your goals this week:

- Complete 5-6 sessions of recumbent cardio (25-30 minutes each)
- Work in Base Pace to Maximal Steady State (60-80% max HR or RPE 5-7)
- Include two interval sessions (increased from one)
- Complete 2 strength training sessions (continued progression)
- Hit 30 minutes continuous by end of week
- Notice improved recovery between sessions

What you'll feel: Week 6 often feels better than Week 5. The initial Phase 2 adjustment is done. Your body knows what's expected. The intervals don't feel as shocking. Thirty minutes still requires mental endurance, but physically you're capable. Many people report feeling genuinely stronger this week.

Daily Workout Schedule

Day 1: Monday

- Equipment: Recumbent bike
- Duration: 25 minutes continuous
- Intensity: Base Pace (60-70% max HR or RPE 5-6)
- Instructions: Solid steady state work to start the week.

Day 2: Tuesday

- Equipment: Rowing machine (or alternate)
- Duration: 25 minutes with intervals
- Intensity: Base Pace with Maximal Steady State intervals
- Instructions: **Interval Session**
    - Warm up 5 minutes
    - Minutes 6-20: Alternate 2 minutes Base Pace, 1 minute Maximal Steady State
    - Complete 5 intervals
    - Cool down 5 minutes

- Strength Training Session 1

Day 3: Wednesday

- Equipment: Recumbent bike
- Duration: 28 minutes continuous
- Intensity: Maximal Steady State (70-80% max HR or RPE 6-7)
- Instructions: Longest session at higher sustained intensity. This is challenging. Check heart rate every 7 minutes.

Day 4: Thursday

- Equipment: Swimming (or alternate)
- Duration: 28 minutes continuous
- Intensity: Base Pace (60-70% max HR or RPE 5-6)
- Instructions: Recovery intensity after yesterday's harder work.
- Strength Training Session 2

Day 5: Friday

- Equipment: Recumbent bike
- Duration: 30 minutes with intervals
- Intensity: Base Pace with Maximal Steady State intervals
- Instructions: **Interval Session**
    - Warm up 5 minutes
    - Minutes 6-25: Alternate 2 minutes Base Pace, 1 minute Maximal Steady State
    - Complete 6-7 intervals
    - Cool down 5 minutes
- First 30-minute session. Break into six 5-minute blocks mentally.

Day 6: Saturday

- Equipment: Your choice
- Duration: 30 minutes continuous
- Intensity: Base Pace to Maximal Steady State (65-75% max HR or RPE 5-7)
- Instructions: Final session of Week 6. Thirty continuous minutes. You've built to this.

Day 7: Sunday

- Rest Day

Strength Training Progression

Week 6 Strength Routine (Days 2 and 4):

All Phase 1 exercises continue with increased reps:

- Supine Leg Marches: 25 each leg
- Resistance Band Knee Extensions: 15-18 each leg
- Glute Bridges: 18
- Dead Bugs: 15 each side
- Calf Pumps: 35
- Side-Lying Leg Lifts: 15-18 each leg
- Supine Hip Abduction: 18
- Single-Leg Glute Bridge: 8-10 each leg
- Supine Bicycle Crunches: 24 total

NEW: Resistance Band Pull-Aparts

- Lie on back or sit upright, hold resistance band at chest level, arms extended
- Pull band apart by moving hands out to sides, squeezing shoulder blades together
- Return slowly
- Repetitions: 12-15
- What it works: Upper back, posture muscles (important for upright positioning)

Daily Tracking Logs

Day 1: Date ____________

Equipment: ____________________ Duration: _____ HR Start/Mid/End: //_____

RPE: _____ During (1-10): _____ After (1-10): _____ Next AM (1-10): _____

Notes:

Day 2: Date ____________ (Intervals)

Equipment: ____________________ Duration: _____ Peak interval HR: _____

RPE intervals: _____ During (1-10): _____ After (1-10): _____ Next AM (1-10): _____

Strength: [ ] Completed

Notes:

____

Day 3: Date ____________

Equipment: ____________________ Duration: _____ HR Start/Mid/End: //_____

RPE: _____ During (1-10): _____ After (1-10): _____ Next AM (1-10): _____

Notes:

____

Day 4: Date ____________

Equipment: ____________________ Duration: _____ HR Start/Mid/End: //_____

RPE: _____ During (1-10): _____ After (1-10): _____ Next AM (1-10): _____

Strength: [ ] Completed

Notes:

____

Day 5: Date ____________ (Intervals, 30 minutes)

Equipment: ____________________ Duration: _____ Peak interval HR: _____

RPE intervals: _____ During (1-10): _____ After (1-10): _____ Next AM (1-10): _____

How 30 minutes felt:

____

Notes:

____

Day 6: Date ____________

Equipment: ____________________ Duration: _____ HR Start/Mid/End: //_____

RPE: _____ During (1-10): _____ After (1-10): _____ Next AM (1-10): _____

Notes:

Week 6 Reflection

Sessions completed: _____ out of 6 cardio, _____ out of 2 strength

Total cardio minutes this week: _____ minutes

How this week compared to Week 5:

[ ] Easier [ ] About the same [ ] Harder

How 30-minute sessions felt:

Improvements I notice from Week 1:

Confidence level (1-10): _____

Week 7

You're three-quarters through Phase 2. This week stays at 25-30 minutes but increases the proportion of time you spend at Maximal Steady State. You're building the capacity to sustain higher intensities for longer periods. This is the cardiovascular fitness that will make upright exercise possible in Phase 3.

Week 7 Overview

Your goals this week:

- Complete 5-6 sessions of recumbent cardio (25-30 minutes each)
- Spend more time in Maximal Steady State (70-80% max HR or RPE 6-7)
- Include two interval sessions with longer work periods
- Complete 2 strength training sessions
- Maintain quality through full duration
- Notice improved tolerance to sustained intensity

What you'll feel: This week requires focus. Spending 15-20 minutes of a 30-minute session in Maximal Steady State is real work. You should feel like you're exercising. Breathing harder. Sweating more. Heart rate elevated but controlled. This is appropriate. You're building fitness, not just moving gently.

Daily Workout Schedule

Day 1: Monday

- Equipment: Recumbent bike
- Duration: 25 minutes continuous
- Intensity: Maximal Steady State (70-80% max HR or RPE 6-7)
- Instructions: Full session at higher intensity. Sustainable but challenging.

Day 2: Tuesday

- Equipment: Rowing machine (or alternate)
- Duration: 28 minutes with intervals
- Intensity: Maximal Steady State with brief peaks
- Instructions: **Extended Interval Session**
    - Warm up 5 minutes Base Pace
    - Minutes 6-23: Alternate 3 minutes Maximal Steady State, 1 minute Recovery
    - Complete 4-5 intervals (longer work periods than previous weeks)

    - Cool down 5 minutes
- Strength Training Session 1

Day 3: Wednesday

- Equipment: Recumbent bike
- Duration: 30 minutes continuous
- Intensity: Base Pace to Maximal Steady State (65-75% max HR or RPE 5-7)
- Instructions: Steady work, gradually increasing intensity throughout. Start at Base Pace, finish at Maximal Steady State.

Day 4: Thursday

- Equipment: Swimming (or alternate)
- Duration: 30 minutes continuous
- Intensity: Base Pace (60-70% max HR or RPE 5-6)
- Instructions: Recovery session. Lower intensity, full duration.
- Strength Training Session 2

Day 5: Friday

- Equipment: Recumbent bike
- Duration: 30 minutes with intervals
- Intensity: Maximal Steady State with peaks
- Instructions: **Extended Interval Session**
    - Warm up 5 minutes
    - Minutes 6-25: Alternate 3 minutes Maximal Steady State, 1 minute Recovery
    - Complete 5 intervals
    - Cool down 5 minutes

Day 6: Saturday

- Equipment: Your choice
- Duration: 30 minutes continuous
- Intensity: Maximal Steady State (70-80% max HR or RPE 6-7)
- Instructions: Final session of Week 7. Full duration at sustained higher intensity. This is your peak cardiovascular work while still recumbent.

Day 7: Sunday

- Rest Day

Strength Training Progression

Week 7 Strength Routine (Days 2 and 4):

All previous exercises continue with max Phase 2 reps:

- Supine Leg Marches: 30 each leg
- Resistance Band Knee Extensions: 20 each leg
- Glute Bridges: 20
- Dead Bugs: 18 each side
- Calf Pumps: 40
- Side-Lying Leg Lifts: 20 each leg
- Supine Hip Abduction: 20
- Single-Leg Glute Bridge: 10-12 each leg
- Supine Bicycle Crunches: 30 total
- Resistance Band Pull-Aparts: 15-18

NEW: Prone Back Extensions

- Lie face down, arms at sides or extended overhead
- Lift chest and shoulders off surface, squeezing shoulder blades
- Hold 2 seconds
- Lower slowly
- Repetitions: 10-12
- What it works: Lower back, spinal erectors (critical for upright posture)

Daily Tracking Logs

Day 1: Date ____________

Equipment: ____________________ Duration: _____ HR Start/Mid/End: //_____

RPE: _____ During (1-10): _____ After (1-10): _____ Next AM (1-10): _____

How sustained Maximal Steady State felt: ______________________________________

Notes:

____

Day 2: Date ____________ (Extended Intervals)

Equipment: ____________________ Duration: _____ Peak interval HR: _____

RPE intervals: _____ During (1-10): _____ After (1-10): _____ Next AM (1-10): _____

How 3-minute work intervals felt: ____

Strength: [ ] Completed

Notes:

____

Day 3: Date ____________

Equipment: ____________________ Duration: _____ HR Start/Mid/End: //_____

RPE: _____ During (1-10): _____ After (1-10): _____ Next AM (1-10): _____

Notes:

____

Day 4: Date ____________

Equipment: ____________________ Duration: _____ HR Start/Mid/End: //_____

RPE: _____ During (1-10): _____ After (1-10): _____ Next AM (1-10): _____

Strength: [ ] Completed

Notes:

____

Day 5: Date ____________ (Extended Intervals)

Equipment: ____________________ Duration: _____ Peak interval HR: _____

RPE intervals: _____ During (1-10): _____ After (1-10): _____ Next AM (1-10): _____

Notes:

____

Day 6: Date ____________

Equipment: ____________________ Duration: _____ HR Start/Mid/End: //_____

RPE: _____ During (1-10): _____ After (1-10): _____ Next AM (1-10): _____

Notes:

Week 7 Reflection

Sessions completed: _____ out of 6 cardio, _____ out of 2 strength

Total cardio minutes this week: _____ minutes

Average intensity this week compared to previous weeks:

[ ] Higher [ ] About the same [ ] Lower

How I'm handling sustained Maximal Steady State work:

Confidence level (1-10): _____

Week 8

Final week of Phase 2. You've built from 20 minutes to 30 minutes. You've progressed from Recovery Zone to sustained Maximal Steady State. You've mastered intervals. This week confirms you're ready for the next big step: transitioning to upright exercise in Phase 3. Finish Phase 2 strong.

Week 8 Overview

Your goals this week:

- Complete 5-6 sessions of recumbent cardio (28-30 minutes each)
- Maintain work in Maximal Steady State (70-80% max HR or RPE 6-7)
- Include two interval sessions
- Complete 2 strength training sessions (peak Phase 2 load)
- Successfully complete Phase 2 without setbacks
- Prepare mentally and physically for upright transition

What you'll feel: This week should feel strong. You've adapted to the Phase 2 demands. Thirty minutes at Maximal Steady State is challenging but doable. Your recovery between sessions is faster than it was in Week 5. You might feel legitimately fit for the first time in years. That's real. You've reconditioned your cardiovascular system.

Daily Workout Schedule

Day 1: Monday

- Equipment: Recumbent bike
- Duration: 28 minutes continuous
- Intensity: Maximal Steady State (70-80% max HR or RPE 6-7)
- Instructions: Strong steady state work.

Day 2: Tuesday

- Equipment: Rowing machine (or alternate)
- Duration: 30 minutes with intervals
- Intensity: Maximal Steady State with peaks
- Instructions: **Peak Interval Session**
    - Warm up 5 minutes
    - Minutes 6-25: Alternate 3 minutes Maximal Steady State, 1 minute Recovery
    - Complete 5 intervals

    - Cool down 5 minutes
- Strength Training Session 1

Day 3: Wednesday

- Equipment: Recumbent bike
- Duration: 30 minutes continuous
- Intensity: Maximal Steady State (70-80% max HR or RPE 6-7)
- Instructions: Full duration at sustained intensity. This should feel challenging but manageable.

Day 4: Thursday

- Equipment: Swimming (or alternate)
- Duration: 30 minutes continuous
- Intensity: Base Pace to Maximal Steady State (65-75% max HR or RPE 5-7)
- Instructions: Moderate intensity, full duration.
- Strength Training Session 2

Day 5: Friday

- Equipment: Recumbent bike
- Duration: 30 minutes with intervals
- Intensity: Maximal Steady State with peaks
- Instructions: **Peak Interval Session**
    - Warm up 5 minutes
    - Minutes 6-25: Alternate 3 minutes Maximal Steady State, 1 minute Recovery
    - Complete 5 intervals
    - Cool down 5 minutes

Day 6: Saturday

- Equipment: Your choice
- Duration: 30 minutes continuous
- Intensity: Maximal Steady State (70-80% max HR or RPE 6-7)
- Instructions: Final recumbent session before transitioning to upright in Phase 3. This is your Phase 2 graduation. Thirty continuous minutes at Maximal Steady State on your preferred equipment. Make it count.

Day 7: Sunday

- Rest Day: Celebrate Phase 2 completion. Prepare for Phase 3's upright challenge.

Strength Training Peak

Week 8 represents maximum load for Phase 2 before transitioning to standing exercises in Phase 3.

Week 8 Strength Routine (Days 2 and 4):

All exercises at peak reps:

- Supine Leg Marches: 30 each leg
- Resistance Band Knee Extensions: 20 each leg
- Glute Bridges: 20
- Dead Bugs: 20 each side
- Calf Pumps: 50
- Side-Lying Leg Lifts: 20 each leg
- Supine Hip Abduction: 20
- Single-Leg Glute Bridge: 12-15 each leg
- Supine Bicycle Crunches: 40 total
- Resistance Band Pull-Aparts: 20
- Prone Back Extensions: 15

Daily Tracking Logs

Day 1: Date ____________

Equipment: ____________________ Duration: _____ HR Start/Mid/End: //_____

RPE: _____ During (1-10): _____ After (1-10): _____ Next AM (1-10): _____

Notes:

____

Day 2: Date ____________ (Intervals)

Equipment: ____________________ Duration: _____ Peak interval HR: _____

RPE intervals: _____ During (1-10): _____ After (1-10): _____ Next AM (1-10): _____

Strength: [ ] Completed

Notes:

____

Day 3: Date ____________

Equipment: ____________________ Duration: _____ HR Start/Mid/End: //_____

RPE: _____ During (1-10): _____ After (1-10): _____ Next AM (1-10): _____

Notes:

____

Day 4: Date ____________

Equipment: ____________________ Duration: _____ HR Start/Mid/End: //_____

RPE: _____ During (1-10): _____ After (1-10): _____ Next AM (1-10): _____

Strength: [ ] Completed

Notes:

____

Day 5: Date ____________ (Intervals)

Equipment: ____________________ Duration: _____ Peak interval HR: _____

RPE intervals: _____ During (1-10): _____ After (1-10): _____ Next AM (1-10): _____

Notes:

____

Day 6: Date ____________ (Phase 2 Completion)

Equipment: ____________________ Duration: _____ HR Start/Mid/End: //_____

RPE: _____ During (1-10): _____ After (1-10): _____ Next AM (1-10): _____

How I feel completing Phase 2:

____

____

Notes:

____

Phase 2 Complete Assessment

Total sessions completed in Phase 2: _____ out of 24 cardio, _____ out of 8 strength

Total cardio minutes in Phase 2: _____ minutes

Measurements to retake:

Lying heart rate today: _____ **Week 4 (end Phase 1):** _____ **Baseline:** _____

Standing heart rate (1 minute): _____ **Week 4:** _____ **Baseline:** _____

Standing heart rate (3 minutes): _____ **Week 4:** _____ **Baseline:** _____

Standing tolerance time: _____ **Week 4:** _____ **Baseline:** _____

Changes from Week 4 to Week 8:

____

____

Physical changes I notice:

Cardiovascular endurance: ____

____

Strength:

____

____

Daily symptoms:

____

____

Standing tolerance: ____

____

Most significant accomplishment from Phase 2:

How I feel about starting upright exercise in Phase 3:

[ ] Excited and ready [ ] Nervous but willing [ ] Scared [ ] Not ready yet

If not ready yet, what concerns me: ____

What I've learned about managing my POTS through exercise:

Confidence going into Phase 3 (1-10): _____

PHASE 3: TRANSITIONING UPRIGHT (Weeks 9-12)

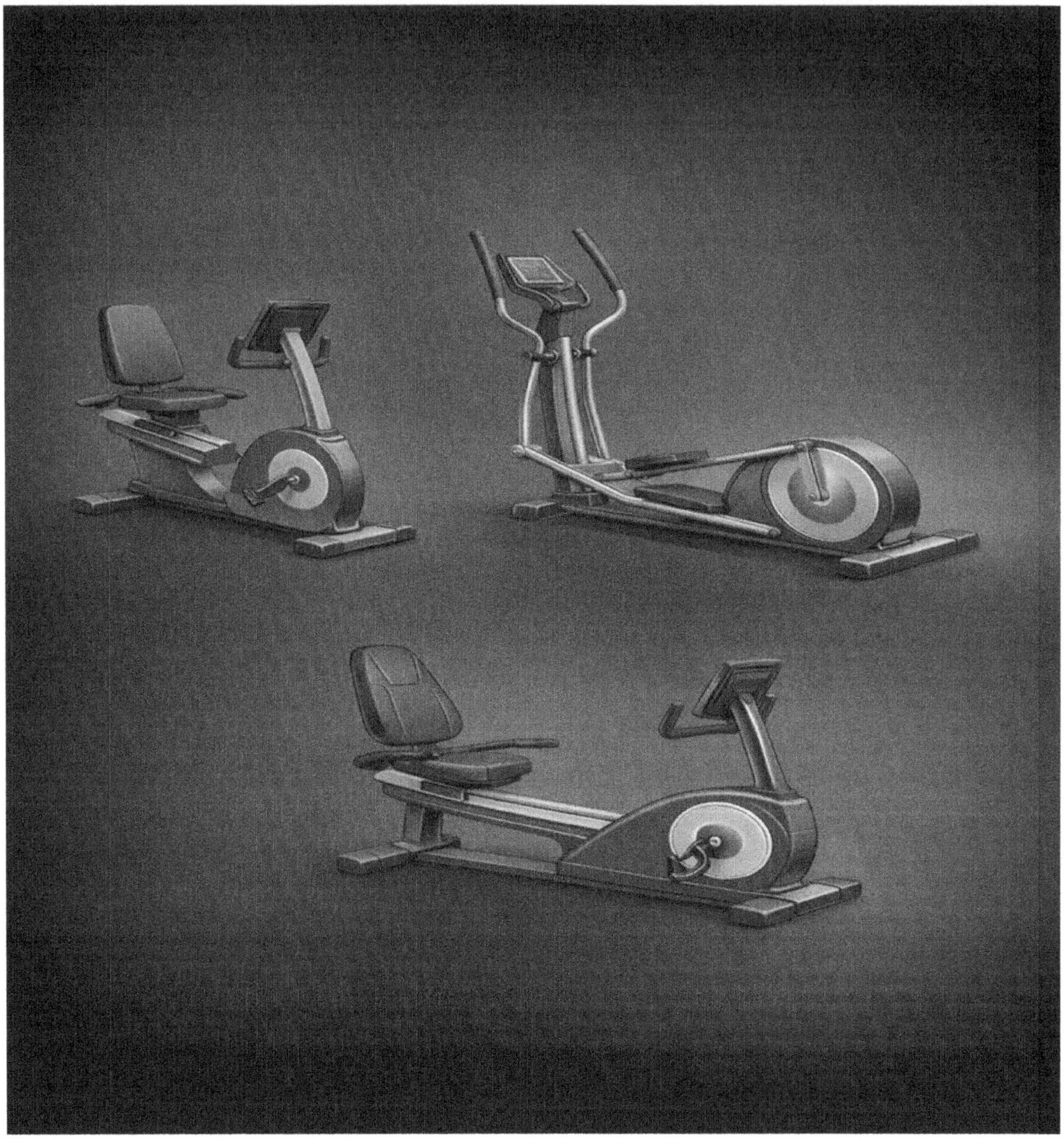

The Critical Shift

You've spent eight weeks building cardiovascular fitness while recumbent. Your heart is larger. Your blood volume is higher. Your muscles are stronger. Now comes the biggest challenge of this program: transitioning to upright exercise. Phase 3 introduces standing exercise gradually, starting in Week 10. You'll learn to manage the orthostatic stress of being upright while exercising. Duration increases to 25-35 minutes. Intensity stays challenging. This phase separates those who complete the protocol from those who don't. Stay consistent. Trust your preparation. Your body is ready for this even when your brain doubts it.

Week 9

Final week of all-recumbent exercise. Week 10 begins the upright transition, so this week solidifies your recumbent fitness and prepares you mentally for the challenge ahead. You'll work in the 28-30 minute range at Maximal Steady State, plus add one longer 35-minute endurance session.

Week 9 Overview

Your goals this week:

- Complete 5-6 sessions of recumbent cardio (28-35 minutes)
- Maintain Maximal Steady State intensity (70-80% max HR or RPE 6-7)
- Complete one 35-minute endurance session
- Complete 2 strength training sessions
- Prepare mentally for upright transition next week
- Finish recumbent-only training on a high note

What you'll feel: This week should feel strong. You're peaking in your recumbent fitness. The 35-minute session is your longest yet, but your body can handle it. Mentally prepare yourself for next week's upright challenge. Upright exercise will feel different, harder, more symptomatic initially. That's expected. The work you're doing this week is building the reserve that makes upright possible.

Daily Workout Schedule

Day 1: Monday

- Equipment: Recumbent bike
- Duration: 28 minutes continuous
- Intensity: Maximal Steady State (70-80% max HR or RPE 6-7)
- Instructions: Strong work to start the week.

Day 2: Tuesday

- Equipment: Rowing machine (or alternate)
- Duration: 30 minutes with intervals
- Intensity: Maximal Steady State with brief peaks
- Instructions: Standard interval session from Phase 2
- Strength Training Session 1

Day 3: Wednesday

- Equipment: Recumbent bike
- Duration: 35 minutes continuous
- Intensity: Base Pace to Maximal Steady State (65-75% max HR or RPE 5-7)
- Instructions: **Longest recumbent session of entire program**. Thirty-five continuous minutes. Start at moderate intensity, build to Maximal Steady State, finish strong. This proves you can sustain extended effort. Break into seven 5-minute blocks mentally.

Day 4: Thursday

- Equipment: Swimming (or alternate)
- Duration: 30 minutes continuous
- Intensity: Base Pace (60-70% max HR or RPE 5-6)
- Instructions: Recovery session after yesterday's long effort.
- Strength Training Session 2

Day 5: Friday

- Equipment: Recumbent bike
- Duration: 30 minutes continuous
- Intensity: Maximal Steady State (70-80% max HR or RPE 6-7)
- Instructions: Solid sustained effort.

Day 6: Saturday

- Equipment: Your choice
- Duration: 30 minutes continuous
- Intensity: Maximal Steady State (70-80% max HR or RPE 6-7)
- Instructions: Final all-recumbent session. Next week you begin upright. Finish this phase knowing you've built the fitness needed for what comes next.

Day 7: Sunday

- Rest Day

Strength Training

Continue Phase 2 peak routine at maximum reps to maintain strength going into upright transition.

Daily Tracking Logs

Day 1: Date ____________

Equipment: _____________ Duration: _____ HR Start/Mid/End: //_____

RPE: _____ During (1-10): _____ After (1-10): _____ Next AM (1-10): _____

Notes:

____

Day 2: Date ____________

Equipment: __________ Duration: _____ HR Start/Mid/End: //_____

RPE: _____ During (1-10): _____ After (1-10): _____ Next AM (1-10): _____

Strength: [ ] Completed

Notes:

____

Day 3: Date ____________ (35 minutes)

Equipment: _____________ Duration: _____ HR Start/Mid/End: //_____

RPE: _____ During (1-10): _____ After (1-10): _____ Next AM (1-10): _____

How 35 continuous minutes felt:

____

____

Notes:

____

Day 4: Date ____________

Equipment: _______________ Duration: _____ HR Start/Mid/End: //_____

RPE: _____ During (1-10): _____ After (1-10): _____ Next AM (1-10): _____

Strength: [ ] Completed

Notes:

Day 5: Date _____________

Equipment: _______________ Duration: _____ HR Start/Mid/End: //_____

RPE: _____ During (1-10): _____ After (1-10): _____ Next AM (1-10): _____

Notes:

Day 6: Date _____________

Equipment: ______________ Duration: _____ HR Start/Mid/End: //_____

RPE: _____ During (1-10): _____ After (1-10): _____ Next AM (1-10): _____

Completing all-recumbent training:

Notes:

Preparing for Upright Exercise

Next week you begin upright cardio. Here's what to expect and how to prepare.

What changes in Week 10:

- You'll add 5-10 minutes of upright exercise (upright bike or elliptical) to some sessions
- Your heart rate will spike higher when upright even at same effort level
- You'll feel more symptoms initially (lightheadedness, fatigue, heart racing)
- This is normal and temporary

- You'll continue recumbent work as the base, adding upright as supplement

How to manage the transition:

- Wear compression garments for all sessions going forward
- Increase sodium and fluid intake on upright exercise days
- Move slowly when transitioning from seated to standing
- Stop immediately if you feel faint or extremely symptomatic
- Expect that upright will feel hard—that doesn't mean you can't do it
- Progress slowly with upright time

My Preparation:

Compression garments: [ ] Ready [ ] Need to obtain

Extra sodium strategy for upright days: ____

____

How I'm feeling about starting upright: [ ] Ready [ ] Nervous [ ] Scared

What concerns me most:

____

____

What I'll remind myself when upright feels hard: ______________________________

____

____

Week 9 Reflection

Sessions completed: _____ out of 6 cardio, _____ out of 2 strength

Total cardio minutes this week: _____ minutes

Longest single session: _____ minutes

How I feel completing nine weeks:

____

Physical changes from Week 1 to Week 9:

Confidence level (1-10): _____

I'm ready for upright because:

Week 10

This is it. The week you've been building toward. You're adding upright exercise. Today you'll stand while exercising for the first time in this program. It will feel hard. Your heart rate will spike. You might feel lightheaded. This is expected. Your cardiovascular system knows how to handle exercise now—it just needs to learn how to do it while fighting gravity. Start small. Progress slowly. Trust the process.

Week 10 Overview

Your goals this week:

- Complete 5-6 cardio sessions (25-30 minutes each)
- Include 5-10 minutes of upright exercise in 3 sessions
- Continue recumbent as base (15-20 minutes) before upright segments
- Complete 2 strength training sessions (adding standing exercises)
- Successfully tolerate upright segments without crashing
- Build confidence in upright capacity

What you'll feel: Upright exercise feels dramatically different than recumbent. Your heart rate will be 20-40 beats higher for the same perceived effort. You'll feel your symptoms more. Your legs might feel shaky. You might feel lightheaded. All normal. The recumbent portion should feel easy now—good. That allows you to push through the harder upright work.

Equipment needed: Upright stationary bike or elliptical machine. These are safer than treadmill for initial upright work because you can hold onto handles. Continue access to recumbent equipment.

Critical success factors:

- Wear compression garments for all sessions
- Pre-load with sodium and fluids
- Move slowly when transitioning to standing
- Stop if symptoms become severe (9-10 on symptom scale)
- Celebrate completing even 5 minutes upright

Daily Workout Schedule

Day 1: Monday

- Recumbent warm-up: 20 minutes at Base Pace

- **NEW: Upright segment**: 5 minutes on upright bike or elliptical
    - Start very slowly, low resistance
    - Target heart rate: Recovery to Base Pace (50-65% max HR)
    - If heart rate goes above 75% max, slow down immediately
    - Normal for heart rate to be 20-30 beats higher than recumbent
- Cool down: 5 minutes recumbent
- **Total duration: 30 minutes** (20 recumbent, 5 upright, 5 cool down)

Day 2: Tuesday

- Recumbent only: 30 minutes at Maximal Steady State
- Strength Training Session 1 (adding standing exercises)

Day 3: Wednesday

- Recumbent warm-up: 18 minutes at Base Pace
- **Upright segment**: 7 minutes on upright bike or elliptical
    - Low to moderate resistance
    - Target heart rate: Base Pace (60-70% max HR)
    - Check heart rate at 3 minutes and 6 minutes
    - Second upright session should feel slightly easier than Monday
- Cool down: 5 minutes recumbent
- **Total duration: 30 minutes**

Day 4: Thursday

- Recumbent only: 30 minutes at Base Pace
- This is recovery from upright work
- Strength Training Session 2

Day 5: Friday

- Recumbent warm-up: 18 minutes at Base Pace
- **Upright segment**: 10 minutes on upright bike or elliptical
    - Moderate resistance
    - Target heart rate: Base Pace (60-70% max HR)
    - Longest upright session yet
    - Break into two 5-minute blocks mentally
    - You can do this
- Cool down: 7 minutes recumbent
- **Total duration: 35 minutes**

Day 6: Saturday

- Recumbent only: 30 minutes at Maximal Steady State
- Solid work to finish Week 10

Day 7: Sunday

- Rest Day

Adding Standing Strength Exercises

Week 10 introduces standing exercises to strength training. These build the leg and core stability needed for upright cardio.

Week 10 Strength Routine (Days 2 and 4):

Continue key lying exercises:

- Glute Bridges: 20
- Dead Bugs: 20 each side
- Calf Pumps: 50
- Single-Leg Glute Bridge: 15 each leg

NEW: Standing Exercises

Standing March in Place

- Stand holding onto chair or wall for support
- March in place, lifting knees to comfortable height
- Duration: 1 minute continuous
- What it works: Hip flexors, cardiovascular tolerance to standing

Standing Calf Raises

- Stand with feet hip-width, holding support
- Rise up onto toes
- Hold 1 second
- Lower slowly
- Repetitions: 15
- What it works: Calf strength and pump function

Standing Hip Abduction

- Stand holding support

- Lift one leg out to side, keeping leg straight
- Hold 1 second
- Lower slowly
- Complete one side, then other
- Repetitions: 10 each leg
- What it works: Hip stabilizers for upright balance

Wall Squats

- Lean back against wall
- Feet hip-width, about 12 inches from wall
- Slide down wall until knees at 45-60 degree angle (NOT full squat)
- Hold 10-15 seconds
- Slide back up
- Repetitions: 5-8
- What it works: Quads, glutes, overall leg strength

Standing Core Bracing

- Stand with good posture
- Contract abs as if bracing for a punch
- Hold 10 seconds while breathing normally
- Relax
- Repetitions: 5
- What it works: Core stability while upright

Managing Upright Exercise

Before starting upright segment:

- Put on compression garments if not already wearing
- Drink 8-12 oz fluid with electrolytes
- Set up equipment at easiest settings
- Have water bottle within reach
- Plan to start very slowly

During upright exercise:

- Check heart rate frequently (every 2-3 minutes)
- Monitor symptoms actively
- If lightheaded, slow down immediately but stay upright if safe
- If extremely symptomatic (seeing spots, feeling faint), sit down immediately

- Focus on completing prescribed time, not on intensity

After upright exercise:

- Don't stop moving abruptly—transition to slow recumbent work
- Cool down minimum 5 minutes before stopping completely
- Stay seated 5-10 minutes after stopping exercise
- Drink 16-24 oz fluid with sodium
- Monitor symptoms for next hour

Daily Tracking Logs

Day 1: Date ____________ (First Upright)

Recumbent: _____ minutes Equipment: ____________________

Upright segment: _____ minutes Equipment: ____________________

Recumbent HR: _____ Upright HR start: _____ Upright HR end: _____

RPE upright: _____ During (1-10): _____ After (1-10): _____ Next AM (1-10): _____

Symptoms during upright (rate 1-10):

Lightheadedness: _____ Nausea: _____ Heart racing: _____ Shakiness: _____

How first upright session felt:

Strength: [ ] Completed (standing exercises)

Notes:

Day 2: Date ____________

Recumbent only: _____ minutes HR: //_____

RPE: _____ During (1-10): _____ After (1-10): _____ Next AM (1-10): _____

Strength: [ ] Completed

Notes:

Day 3: Date ____________ (Second Upright)

Recumbent: _____ minutes **Upright:** _____ minutes

Recumbent HR: _____ Upright HR start: _____ Upright HR end: _____

RPE upright: _____ During (1-10): _____ After (1-10): _____ Next AM (1-10): _____

Symptoms during upright: Lightheadedness: _____ Nausea: _____ Heart racing: _____ Shakiness: _____

How second upright session compared to first:

Notes:

Day 4: Date ____________

Recumbent only: _____ minutes HR: //_____

RPE: _____ During (1-10): _____ After (1-10): _____ Next AM (1-10): _____

Strength: [ ] Completed

Notes:

Day 5: Date ____________ (Longest Upright)

Recumbent: _____ minutes **Upright:** _____ minutes

Recumbent HR: _____ Upright HR start: _____ Upright HR mid: _____ Upright HR end: _____

RPE upright: _____ During (1-10): _____ After (1-10): _____ Next AM (1-10): _____

Symptoms during upright: Lightheadedness: _____ Nausea: _____ Heart racing: _____ Shakiness: _____

How 10 minutes upright felt:

Notes:

Day 6: Date ____________

Recumbent only: _____ minutes HR: //_____

RPE: _____ During (1-10): _____ After (1-10): _____ Next AM (1-10): _____

Notes:

Week 10 Reflection

Total upright minutes this week: _____ minutes (across 3 sessions)

Upright sessions completed: _____ out of 3 prescribed

How upright exercise felt compared to my expectations:

Biggest challenge with upright:

What helped me get through upright segments:

Symptoms during upright (which were most prominent):

Did I crash this week? [ ] No [ ] Yes (if yes, describe: ______________________)

Confidence level with upright (1-10): _____

What I need to work on for Week 11:

I'm proud of myself for:

Week 11

You survived your first week of upright exercise. You proved you can do it. This week increases upright time to 10-15 minutes per session across more sessions. You're building tolerance to standing while exercising. It should feel slightly easier this week than last week, though still challenging. Keep going.

Week 11 Overview

Your goals this week:

- Complete 5-6 cardio sessions (28-35 minutes each)
- Include 10-15 minutes of upright exercise in 4 sessions (increased from 3)
- Continue recumbent as warm-up and cool-down
- Complete 2 strength training sessions (progressing standing work)
- Increase upright tolerance with less symptom intensity
- Build confidence and consistency with standing exercise

What you'll feel: Upright should feel more doable this week. Your nervous system is adapting. Heart rate won't spike quite as high. Symptoms should be less intense. You'll still feel the challenge, but it's manageable. If you're not seeing improvement in how upright feels, check: Are you wearing compression? Getting enough sodium? Staying adequately hydrated? Moving slowly when transitioning to standing?

Daily Workout Schedule

Day 1: Monday

- Recumbent warm-up: 15 minutes at Base Pace
- Upright segment: 10 minutes on upright bike or elliptical
- Cool down: 5 minutes recumbent
- **Total: 30 minutes**

Day 2: Tuesday

- Recumbent warm-up: 15 minutes at Base Pace
- Upright segment: 12 minutes on upright bike or elliptical
- Cool down: 8 minutes recumbent
- **Total: 35 minutes**
- Strength Training Session 1

Day 3: Wednesday

- Recumbent only: 30 minutes at Maximal Steady State
- Recovery from two upright days

Day 4: Thursday

- Recumbent warm-up: 15 minutes at Base Pace
- Upright segment: 15 minutes on upright bike or elliptical
- Cool down: 5 minutes recumbent
- **Total: 35 minutes** (longest upright yet)
- Strength Training Session 2

Day 5: Friday

- Recumbent only: 30 minutes at Base Pace
- Recovery day

Day 6: Saturday

- Recumbent warm-up: 13 minutes at Base Pace
- Upright segment: 15 minutes on upright bike or elliptical
- Cool down: 7 minutes recumbent
- **Total: 35 minutes**

Day 7: Sunday

- Rest Day

Strength Training Progression

Week 11 Strength Routine (Days 2 and 4):

Continue lying exercises (reduced volume to accommodate standing work):

- Glute Bridges: 15
- Dead Bugs: 15 each side
- Single-Leg Glute Bridge: 12 each leg

Progressed Standing Exercises:

Standing March in Place

- Duration: 2 minutes (increased from 1 minute)

Standing Calf Raises

- Repetitions: 20 (increased from 15)

Standing Hip Abduction

- Repetitions: 12-15 each leg

Wall Squats

- Hold: 15-20 seconds each
- Repetitions: 8-10

Standing Core Bracing

- Hold: 15 seconds each
- Repetitions: 8

NEW: Step-Ups

- Use 4-6 inch step (stair or platform)
- Step up with one foot, bring other foot up
- Step down same way
- Alternate leading leg every 5 reps
- Repetitions: 10 total (5 each leg leading)
- What it works: Leg strength, coordination, mimics upright movement

Daily Tracking Logs

Day 1: Date _____________

Recumbent: _____ min Upright: _____ min Total: _____ min

Upright HR start/mid/end: //_____ RPE upright: _____

During (1-10): _____ After (1-10): _____ Next AM (1-10): _____

Symptoms during upright: Lightheaded: _____ Nausea: _____ Racing: _____ Shaky: _____

Notes:

Day 2: Date _____________

Recumbent: _____ min Upright: _____ min Total: _____ min

Upright HR start/mid/end: //_____ RPE upright: _____

During (1-10): _____ After (1-10): _____ Next AM (1-10): _____

Strength: [ ] Completed

Notes:

Day 3: Date _____________

Recumbent only: _____ min HR: //_____

RPE: _____ During (1-10): _____ After (1-10): _____ Next AM (1-10): _____

Notes:

Day 4: Date _____________ (15 minutes upright)

Recumbent: _____ min Upright: _____ min Total: _____ min

Upright HR start/mid/end: //_____ RPE upright: _____

During (1-10): _____ After (1-10): _____ Next AM (1-10): _____

How 15 minutes upright felt:

Strength: [ ] Completed

Notes:

Day 5: Date ____________

Recumbent only: _____ min HR: //_____

RPE: _____ During (1-10): _____ After (1-10): _____ Next AM (1-10): _____

Notes:

____

Day 6: Date ____________

Recumbent: _____ min Upright: _____ min Total: _____ min

Upright HR start/mid/end: //_____ RPE upright: _____

During (1-10): _____ After (1-10): _____ Next AM (1-10): _____

Notes:

____

Week 11 Reflection

Total upright minutes this week: _____ minutes (across 4 sessions)

How upright felt this week compared to Week 10:

[ ] Easier [ ] About the same [ ] Harder

Improvements I notice in upright tolerance:

____

____

Challenges that remain:

____

____

Confidence level (1-10): _____

____

Week 12

Final week of Phase 3. This week pushes upright time to 15-20 minutes per session. By Saturday, you'll complete 20 continuous minutes of upright exercise—the same duration you did recumbent at end of Phase 1. You've come full circle, but now you're doing it standing. This is massive progress.

Week 12 Overview

Your goals this week:

- Complete 5-6 cardio sessions (30-35 minutes each)
- Include 15-20 minutes of upright exercise in 4-5 sessions
- Successfully complete 20 minutes continuous upright
- Complete 2 strength training sessions (peak standing load)
- Finish Phase 3 strong
- Prepare for Phase 4's all-upright work

What you'll feel: Twenty minutes upright is real work. You'll need mental focus and physical endurance. Your legs might get tired before your cardiovascular system does. Your symptoms should be manageable by now. If upright still feels unbearable, extend Phase 3 by repeating Week 11 before advancing to Week 12. Most people are ready to progress. Trust your tracking data.

Daily Workout Schedule

Day 1: Monday

- Recumbent warm-up: 12 minutes at Base Pace
- Upright segment: 15 minutes on upright bike or elliptical at Base Pace
- Cool down: 8 minutes recumbent
- **Total: 35 minutes**

Day 2: Tuesday

- Recumbent warm-up: 10 minutes
- Upright segment: 18 minutes
- Cool down: 7 minutes recumbent
- **Total: 35 minutes**
- Strength Training Session 1

Day 3: Wednesday

- Recumbent only: 30 minutes at Maximal Steady State
- Recovery intensity

Day 4: Thursday

- Recumbent warm-up: 10 minutes
- Upright segment: 20 minutes on upright bike or elliptical
- Cool down: 5 minutes recumbent
- **Total: 35 minutes** (longest upright yet)
- Strength Training Session 2

Day 5: Friday

- Recumbent warm-up: 15 minutes
- Upright segment: 15 minutes
- Cool down: 5 minutes recumbent
- **Total: 35 minutes**

Day 6: Saturday

- Recumbent warm-up: 10 minutes at Base Pace
- **Upright segment: 20 minutes on upright bike or elliptical at Base Pace to Maximal Steady State**
- Cool down: 5 minutes recumbent
- **Total: 35 minutes**
- This is your Phase 3 graduation: 20 continuous minutes upright

Day 7: Sunday

- Rest Day: Celebrate Phase 3 completion

Strength Training Peak

Week 12 Strength Routine (Days 2 and 4):

Reduced lying work:

- Glute Bridges: 12
- Dead Bugs: 12 each side

Peak Standing Exercises:

Standing March in Place: 3 minutes **Standing Calf Raises:** 25 **Standing Hip Abduction:** 15 each leg **Wall Squats:** 20-30 second holds, 10 reps **Standing Core Bracing:** 20 seconds, 10 reps **Step-Ups:** 15 total (alternating legs)

NEW: Standing Heel-to-Toe Walk

- Walk forward placing heel directly in front of toes
- Arms out for balance
- Focus on slow, controlled movement
- Distance: 10-15 feet, repeat 3-4 times
- What it works: Balance, coordination, ankle stability

Daily Tracking Logs

Day 1: Date ____________

Recumbent: _____ min Upright: _____ min Total: _____ min

Upright HR: //_____ RPE upright: _____

During (1-10): _____ After (1-10): _____ Next AM (1-10): _____

Notes:

____

Day 2: Date ____________

Recumbent: _____ min Upright: _____ min Total: _____ min

Upright HR: //_____ RPE upright: _____

During (1-10): _____ After (1-10): _____ Next AM (1-10): _____

Strength: [ ] Completed

Notes:

____

Day 3: Date ____________

Recumbent only: _____ min HR: //_____

RPE: _____ During (1-10): _____ After (1-10): _____ Next AM (1-10): _____

Notes:

___

Day 4: Date ____________ (20 minutes upright)

Recumbent: _____ min Upright: _____ min Total: _____ min

Upright HR: //_____ RPE upright: _____

During (1-10): _____ After (1-10): _____ Next AM (1-10): _____

How 20 minutes upright felt:

___

___

Strength: [ ] Completed

Notes:

___

Day 5: Date ____________

Recumbent: _____ min Upright: _____ min Total: _____ min

Upright HR: //_____ RPE upright: _____

During (1-10): _____ After (1-10): _____ Next AM (1-10): _____

Notes:

___

Day 6: Date ____________ (Phase 3 Completion)

Recumbent: _____ min Upright: _____ min Total: _____ min

Upright HR: //_____ RPE upright: _____

During (1-10): _____ After (1-10): _____ Next AM (1-10): _____

Completing 20 minutes upright:

____

____

Notes:

____

Phase 3 Complete Assessment

Total upright minutes in Phase 3: _____ minutes

Upright sessions completed: _____ out of 12-15 prescribed

Measurements to retake:

Lying heart rate: _____ **Week 8:** _____ **Baseline:** _____

Standing heart rate (1 min): _____ **Week 8:** _____ **Baseline:** _____

Standing heart rate (3 min): _____ **Week 8:** _____ **Baseline:** _____

Standing tolerance: _____ **Week 8:** _____ **Baseline:** _____

Changes from Week 8 to Week 12:

____

____

How upright exercise evolved from Week 10 to Week 12:

Week 10:

____

Week 12:

____

Difference:

____

Most significant accomplishment from Phase 3:

How I feel about starting all-upright work in Phase 4:

Confidence level (1-10): _____

PHASE 4: UPRIGHT MASTERY (Weeks 13-16)

Reclaiming Function

You did it. You transitioned to upright exercise. You can now do 20 minutes standing while exercising. Phase 4 builds on this foundation. You'll work primarily upright for 30-45 minutes per session. You'll reintroduce intervals while standing. You'll add treadmill walking with incline. By Week 16, you'll be doing exercise that looked impossible 12 weeks ago. This is the home stretch. Finish what you started.

Week 13

First week of primarily upright exercise. You'll do 20-25 minutes upright per session with minimal recumbent warm-up. The focus shifts from "Can I tolerate upright?" to "How much work can I do while upright?" You're building cardiovascular capacity in the position your body needs for real life.

Week 13 Overview

Your goals this week:

- Complete 5-6 cardio sessions (30-40 minutes each)
- Work 20-25 minutes upright per session
- Keep recumbent warm-up brief (5-10 minutes)
- Work in Base Pace to Maximal Steady State zones while upright
- Complete 2 strength training sessions
- Build upright endurance and confidence

What you'll feel: This week requires sustained upright work. Twenty to twenty-five minutes standing while exercising is significant. Your legs will get tired. That's normal—they're working hard to pump blood back to your heart. Compression helps. Taking the last 5-10 minutes at slightly lower intensity is fine. The goal is completing the time upright, not maintaining peak intensity the entire session.

Daily Workout Schedule

Day 1: Monday

- Recumbent warm-up: 5 minutes
- Upright: 20 minutes on upright bike or elliptical at Base Pace
- Cool down: 5 minutes recumbent
- **Total: 30 minutes**

Day 2: Tuesday

- Recumbent warm-up: 5 minutes
- Upright: 25 minutes on upright bike at Base Pace to Maximal Steady State
- Cool down: 5 minutes recumbent
- **Total: 35 minutes**
- Strength Training Session 1

Day 3: Wednesday

- Recumbent warm-up: 10 minutes
- Upright: 20 minutes at Maximal Steady State
- Cool down: 5 minutes recumbent
- **Total: 35 minutes**

Day 4: Thursday

- Recumbent only: 30 minutes at Base Pace
- Recovery from three upright days
- Strength Training Session 2

Day 5: Friday

- Recumbent warm-up: 5 minutes
- Upright: 25 minutes at Base Pace to Maximal Steady State
- Cool down: 5 minutes recumbent
- **Total: 35 minutes**

Day 6: Saturday

- Recumbent warm-up: 5 minutes
- **NEW: Treadmill walking** (flat surface, slow speed)
- Upright: 25 minutes treadmill or continue bike/elliptical
- Cool down: 5 minutes recumbent
- **Total: 35 minutes**

Day 7: Sunday

- Rest Day

Introducing Treadmill Walking

Saturday introduces treadmill walking option. Walking is the most functional upright exercise—it's what you do in daily life.

Treadmill Guidelines:

- Start flat (0% incline)
- Speed: 2.0-2.5 mph initially (slower than normal walking)
- Hold handrails lightly for balance if needed

- Focus on posture: shoulders back, core engaged
- If heart rate goes above Maximal Steady State, slow speed
- Build to comfortable 2.5-3.0 mph before adding incline

When to use treadmill vs bike/elliptical:

- Treadmill: Most functional, best for real-life preparation
- Bike/elliptical: Safer if balance concerns, easier to monitor heart rate

Strength Training

Week 13 Strength Routine (Days 2 and 4):

Minimal lying work:

- Dead Bugs: 15 each side

Primary Standing Focus:

Standing March in Place: 3 minutes **Standing Calf Raises:** 30 **Standing Hip Abduction:** 18 each leg **Wall Squats:** 30-second holds, 10 reps **Standing Core Bracing:** 30 seconds, 8 reps **Step-Ups:** 20 total **Standing Heel-to-Toe Walk:** 15 feet, 5 times

NEW: Standing Resistance Band Rows

- Attach band to stable object at chest height
- Stand holding band handles, arms extended
- Pull handles to sides of chest, squeezing shoulder blades
- Return slowly
- Repetitions: 12-15
- What it works: Upper back, posture, standing stability

Daily Tracking Logs

Day 1: Date _____________

Warmup: _____ min Upright: _____ min Cooldown: _____ min Total: _____ min

Upright HR: //_____ RPE: _____

During (1-10): _____ After (1-10): _____ Next AM (1-10): _____

Notes:

Day 2: Date _____________

Warmup: _____ min Upright: _____ min Cooldown: _____ min Total: _____ min

Upright HR: //_____ RPE: _____

During (1-10): _____ After (1-10): _____ Next AM (1-10): _____

Strength: [ ] Completed

Notes:

Day 3: Date _____________

Warmup: _____ min Upright: _____ min Cooldown: _____ min Total: _____ min

Upright HR: //_____ RPE: _____

During (1-10): _____ After (1-10): _____ Next AM (1-10): _____

Notes:

Day 4: Date _____________

Recumbent only: _____ min HR: //_____

During (1-10): _____ After (1-10): _____ Next AM (1-10): _____

Strength: [ ] Completed

Notes:

Day 5: Date _____________

Warmup: _____ min Upright: _____ min Cooldown: _____ min Total: _____ min

Upright HR: //_____ RPE: _____

During (1-10): _____ After (1-10): _____ Next AM (1-10): _____

Notes:

Day 6: Date _____________ (Treadmill option)

Warmup: _____ min **Upright (treadmill or bike):** _____ min Cooldown: _____ min

If treadmill: Speed: _____ mph Incline: ***% HR: //***

During (1-10): _____ After (1-10): _____ Next AM (1-10): _____

Notes:

Week 13 Reflection

Total upright minutes this week: _____ minutes

How sustained upright work felt:

If I tried treadmill, how it compared to bike/elliptical:

Confidence level (1-10): _____

Week 14

You're getting close to the end. This week increases upright time to 25-30 minutes per session. You'll add incline walking if using treadmill. You'll reintroduce intervals while upright. This is peak cardiovascular work for the entire program.

Week 14 Overview

Your goals this week:

- Complete 5-6 cardio sessions (35-40 minutes each)
- Work 25-30 minutes upright per session
- Include intervals while upright (2 sessions)
- Add treadmill incline if using treadmill
- Complete 2 strength training sessions
- Push intensity while maintaining upright position

What you'll feel: This is hard work. You're doing what healthy, fit people do. Thirty minutes upright at Maximal Steady State with intervals is legitimate exercise. Your POTS symptoms should be minimal during sessions now. If they're not, check your recovery strategies: sodium, hydration, compression, sleep. You've built the capacity. Now you're refining it.

Daily Workout Schedule

Day 1: Monday

- Recumbent warm-up: 5 minutes
- Upright: 25 minutes at Base Pace
- Cool down: 5 minutes recumbent
- **Total: 35 minutes**

Day 2: Tuesday

- Recumbent warm-up: 5 minutes
- **Upright with intervals: 28 minutes**
  - 5 minutes Base Pace
  - Intervals: 2 minutes Maximal Steady State, 2 minutes Base Pace (repeat 6 times)
  - 2 minutes cool down
- Cool down: 5 minutes recumbent
- **Total: 38 minutes**

- Strength Training Session 1

Day 3: Wednesday

- Recumbent warm-up: 5 minutes
- Upright: 30 minutes at Maximal Steady State
- Cool down: 5 minutes recumbent
- **Total: 40 minutes** (longest session yet)

Day 4: Thursday

- Recumbent only: 30 minutes at Base Pace
- Recovery day
- Strength Training Session 2

Day 5: Friday

- Recumbent warm-up: 5 minutes
- **Upright with intervals: 30 minutes**
    - 5 minutes Base Pace
    - Intervals: 2 minutes Maximal Steady State, 2 minutes Base Pace (repeat 6 times)
    - 3 minutes cool down
- Cool down: 5 minutes recumbent
- **Total: 40 minutes**

Day 6: Saturday

- Recumbent warm-up: 5 minutes
- **Upright: 30 minutes treadmill with incline** (or bike/elliptical at higher resistance)
    - If treadmill: Start flat, gradually increase to 3-5% incline
    - Speed: 2.5-3.0 mph
- Cool down: 5 minutes recumbent
- **Total: 40 minutes**

Day 7: Sunday

- Rest Day

Strength Training

Week 14 Strength Routine (Days 2 and 4):

All standing exercises at peak Phase 4 loads:

Standing March in Place: 4 minutes **Standing Calf Raises:** 35 **Standing Hip Abduction:** 20 each leg **Wall Squats:** 45-second holds, 8-10 reps **Step-Ups:** 25 total **Standing Heel-to-Toe Walk:** 20 feet, 6 times **Standing Resistance Band Rows:** 15-18

NEW: Standing Overhead Press

- Hold resistance band handles at shoulder height, band under feet
- Press arms overhead
- Lower slowly
- Repetitions: 10-12
- What it works: Shoulders, core stability while upright

Daily Tracking Logs

Day 1: Date ____________

Warmup: _____ Upright: _____ Cooldown: _____ Total: _____

Upright HR: //_____ RPE: _____

During (1-10): _____ After (1-10): _____ Next AM (1-10): _____

Notes:

____

Day 2: Date ____________ (Intervals)

Warmup: _____ Upright w/intervals: _____ Cooldown: _____ Total: _____

Peak interval HR: _____ RPE intervals: _____

During (1-10): _____ After (1-10): _____ Next AM (1-10): _____

Strength: [ ] Completed

Notes:

____

Day 3: Date ____________

Warmup: _____ Upright: _____ Cooldown: _____ Total: _____

Upright HR: //_____ RPE: _____

During (1-10): _____ After (1-10): _____ Next AM (1-10): _____

Notes:

Day 4: Date _____________

Recumbent only: _____ min

During (1-10): _____ After (1-10): _____ Next AM (1-10): _____

Strength: [ ] Completed

Notes:

Day 5: Date _____________ (Intervals)

Warmup: _____ Upright w/intervals: _____ Cooldown: _____ Total: _____

Peak interval HR: _____ RPE intervals: _____

During (1-10): _____ After (1-10): _____ Next AM (1-10): _____

Notes:

Day 6: Date _____________ (Incline or high resistance)

Warmup: _____ Upright: _____ Cooldown: _____ Total: _____

If treadmill: Speed: _____ Incline: *% HR: //*

During (1-10): _____ After (1-10): _____ Next AM (1-10): _____

Notes:

Week 14 Reflection

Total upright minutes this week: _____ minutes

How intervals felt while upright:

Confidence level (1-10): _____

Week 15

Second-to-last week. You're consolidating everything you've built. This week maintains 30+ minutes upright per session, continues intervals, and adds variety to keep you engaged. You're functioning at a level that seemed impossible 14 weeks ago.

Week 15 Overview

Your goals this week:

- Complete 5-6 cardio sessions (38-45 minutes each)
- Work 30-35 minutes upright per session
- Include 2-3 interval sessions
- Try different upright equipment if available
- Complete 2 strength training sessions
- Finish strong heading into final week

What you'll feel: You should feel capable. Confident. Strong. Thirty-plus minutes upright is no longer frightening—it's just your workout. You can sustain Maximal Steady State. You can handle intervals. Your symptoms are manageable. You've reconditioned your body. This week proves it.

Daily Workout Schedule

Day 1: Monday

- Warmup: 5 minutes recumbent
- Upright: 30 minutes at Maximal Steady State
- Cooldown: 5 minutes
- **Total: 40 minutes**

Day 2: Tuesday

- Warmup: 5 minutes
- Upright with intervals: 32 minutes
    - 8 minutes Base Pace
    - 6 intervals: 2 minutes hard, 2 minutes recovery
    - 8 minutes Base Pace
- Cooldown: 5 minutes
- **Total: 42 minutes**
- Strength Training Session 1

Day 3: Wednesday

- Warmup: 5 minutes
- Upright: 35 minutes at Base Pace to Maximal Steady State
- Cooldown: 5 minutes
- **Total: 45 minutes**

Day 4: Thursday

- Recumbent or light upright: 30 minutes at Base Pace
- Recovery intensity
- Strength Training Session 2

Day 5: Friday

- Warmup: 5 minutes
- Upright with intervals: 32 minutes
- Cooldown: 5 minutes
- **Total: 42 minutes**

Day 6: Saturday

- Warmup: 5 minutes
- **Upright: 35 minutes** (mix of equipment if desired: 15 min treadmill + 20 min bike, or all one type)
- Cooldown: 5 minutes
- **Total: 45 minutes**

Day 7: Sunday

- Rest Day

Strength Training

Continue Week 14 routine at peak loads. Maintain strength as you finish program.

Daily Tracking Logs

Day 1: Date ____________

Warmup: _____ Upright: _____ Cooldown: _____ Total: _____

HR: //_____ RPE: _____

During (1-10): _____ After (1-10): _____ Next AM (1-10): _____

Notes:

Day 2: Date _____________

Total: _____ (with intervals) HR: //_____ RPE: _____

During (1-10): _____ After (1-10): _____ Next AM (1-10): _____

Strength: [ ] Completed

Notes:

Day 3: Date _____________

Warmup: _____ Upright: _____ Cooldown: _____ Total: _____

HR: //_____ RPE: _____

During (1-10): _____ After (1-10): _____ Next AM (1-10): _____

Notes:

Day 4: Date _____________

Exercise: _____ min Type: _____________ HR: //_____

During (1-10): _____ After (1-10): _____ Next AM (1-10): _____

Strength: [ ] Completed

Notes:

Day 5: Date _____________

Total: _____ (with intervals) HR: //_____ RPE: _____

During (1-10): _____ After (1-10): _____ Next AM (1-10): _____

Notes:

____

Day 6: Date ____________

Warmup: _____ Upright: _____ Cooldown: _____ Total: _____

HR: //_____ RPE: _____

During (1-10): _____ After (1-10): _____ Next AM (1-10): _____

Notes:

____

Week 15 Reflection

Total upright minutes this week: _____ minutes

How I feel heading into final week:

____

____

Confidence level (1-10): _____

____

Week 16

Final week. This is it. You've done 15 weeks of consistent work. This week completes the program with 30-45 minutes of upright exercise per session. Saturday is your graduation session: 45 continuous minutes primarily upright at challenging intensity. Finish what you started.

Week 16 Overview

Your goals this week:

- Complete 5-6 cardio sessions (40-45 minutes each)
- Work 30-40 minutes upright per session
- Include challenging intervals
- Complete 45-minute graduation session on Saturday
- Complete 2 strength training sessions
- Finish the 16-week program strong

What you'll feel: You should feel proud. Accomplished. Strong. Capable. You're doing 45 minutes of exercise. You're standing while doing it. Your heart is larger. Your blood volume is higher. Your symptoms are better. You've reconditioned your body through consistency and hard work. This week celebrates that.

Daily Workout Schedule

Day 1: Monday

- Warmup: 5 minutes
- Upright: 30 minutes at Maximal Steady State
- Cooldown: 5 minutes
- **Total: 40 minutes**

Day 2: Tuesday

- Warmup: 5 minutes
- Upright with intervals: 35 minutes
- Cooldown: 5 minutes
- **Total: 45 minutes**
- Strength Training Session 1

Day 3: Wednesday

- Warmup: 5 minutes
- Upright: 35 minutes at Base Pace to Maximal Steady State
- Cooldown: 5 minutes
- **Total: 45 minutes**

Day 4: Thursday

- Light recumbent or easy upright: 30 minutes
- Recovery for graduation session
- Strength Training Session 2

Day 5: Friday

- Warmup: 5 minutes
- Upright: 30 minutes at Base Pace
- Cooldown: 5 minutes
- **Total: 40 minutes**

Day 6: Saturday - GRADUATION SESSION

- Warmup: 5 minutes recumbent at easy pace
- **Upright: 35-40 minutes**
    - First 15 minutes: Base Pace to Maximal Steady State
    - Middle 10-15 minutes: Sustained Maximal Steady State
    - Final 10 minutes: Base Pace, finish strong
- Cooldown: 5-10 minutes recumbent, easy pace
- **Total: 45-50 minutes**
- **This is your final session. Make it count. Celebrate every minute.**

Day 7: Sunday

- Complete Rest Day
- Celebrate completing 16 weeks
- Reflect on your transformation

Strength Training

Continue peak Phase 4 routine. Final two sessions of structured strength training.

Daily Tracking Logs

Day 1: Date ____________

Warmup: _____ Upright: _____ Cooldown: _____ Total: _____

HR: /\/_____ RPE: _____

During (1-10): _____ After (1-10): _____ Next AM (1-10): _____

Notes:

Day 2: Date _____________

Total: _____ (with intervals) HR: /\/_____ RPE: _____

During (1-10): _____ After (1-10): _____ Next AM (1-10): _____

Strength: [ ] Completed

Notes:

Day 3: Date _____________

Warmup: _____ Upright: _____ Cooldown: _____ Total: _____

HR: /\/_____ RPE: _____

During (1-10): _____ After (1-10): _____ Next AM (1-10): _____

Notes:

Day 4: Date _____________

Exercise: _____ min HR: /\/_____

During (1-10): _____ After (1-10): _____ Next AM (1-10): _____

Strength: [ ] Completed

Notes:

Day 5: Date ____________

Warmup: _____ Upright: _____ Cooldown: _____ Total: _____

HR: /\/_____ RPE: _____

During (1-10): _____ After (1-10): _____ Next AM (1-10): _____

Notes:

____

Day 6: Date ____________ 🎓 GRADUATION SESSION 🎓

Warmup: _____ **UPRIGHT: _____** Cooldown: _____ **TOTAL: _____**

HR Start: _____ HR Mid: _____ HR End: _____ Peak HR: _____

RPE: _____ During (1-10): _____ After (1-10): _____ Next AM (1-10): _____

How completing 16 weeks feels:

____

____

____

____

____

What I want to remember about this final session:

____

____

____

____

Notes:

____

____

Program Completion Assessment

Total sessions completed in 16 weeks:

Phase 1: _____ out of 24 cardio, _____ out of 8 strength

Phase 2: _____ out of 24 cardio, _____ out of 8 strength

Phase 3: _____ out of 24 cardio, _____ out of 8 strength

Phase 4: _____ out of 24 cardio, _____ out of 8 strength

TOTAL: _____ out of 96 cardio sessions, _____ out of 32 strength sessions

Total exercise minutes in 16 weeks: _____ minutes

Final Measurements:

Lying heart rate: _____ Baseline (Week 0): _____ Change: _____

Standing HR (1 min): _____ Baseline: _____ Change: _____

Standing HR (3 min): _____ Baseline: _____ Change: _____

Standing tolerance: _____ min **Baseline: _____ Change: _____**

Physical changes over 16 weeks:

Week 1 to Week 16 cardiovascular capacity: ______________________________

____

Symptom changes:

____

____

Standing tolerance: ______________________________

____

Daily function:

____

____

Strength changes:

Activities I can do now that I couldn't do 16 weeks ago:

Most significant moment in this 16-week journey:

Biggest challenge I overcame:

What I learned about my body:

What I learned about myself:

How this changes my life going forward:

What Comes After Week 16

You've completed the reconditioning protocol. Your cardiovascular system has measurably improved. Now you maintain and continue progressing.

Maintenance options:

Option 1: Continue structured exercise

- 4-5 days per week
- 30-45 minutes per session
- Mix of upright cardio and strength training
- Maintain intensity at Base Pace to Maximal Steady State

Option 2: Return to activities you love

- Walking longer distances
- Light hiking
- Swimming for enjoyment
- Dancing
- Playing with kids/pets
- Gardening
- Sports at recreational intensity

Option 3: Progress further

- Increase duration to 45-60 minutes
- Add more intervals
- Increase treadmill incline to 8-10%
- Try jogging intervals if symptoms allow
- Join exercise classes
- Work with trainer for continued progression

Warning signs of deconditioning:

- Exercise starts feeling much harder than it did
- Standing tolerance decreases
- Symptoms worsen to previous levels
- Resting heart rate increases by 10+ beats

- Orthostatic heart rate increase returns to previous levels

If you notice deconditioning: Return to structured exercise 3-4 days per week for 2-4 weeks to rebuild. Don't let yourself return to baseline.

My Plan After Week 16:

I will exercise: _____ days per week

Type of exercise:

____

Duration: _____ minutes per session

My long-term fitness goal: ____

____

Activities I want to return to: ____________________________________

____

How I'll prevent deconditioning: __________________________________

____

____

Date I completed Week 16: ________________

Signature: ______________________________

____

PART 3: TOOLS & TRACKERS

Chapter 4.0: Exercise Library

This is your reference guide. Every exercise prescribed in the 16-week program is detailed here with proper form, common mistakes, and modifications. Use this chapter when you need to check technique or find alternatives. Good form prevents injury and maximizes effectiveness. Take time to learn these exercises correctly before you start the program.

4.1 Recumbent Cardio Exercises

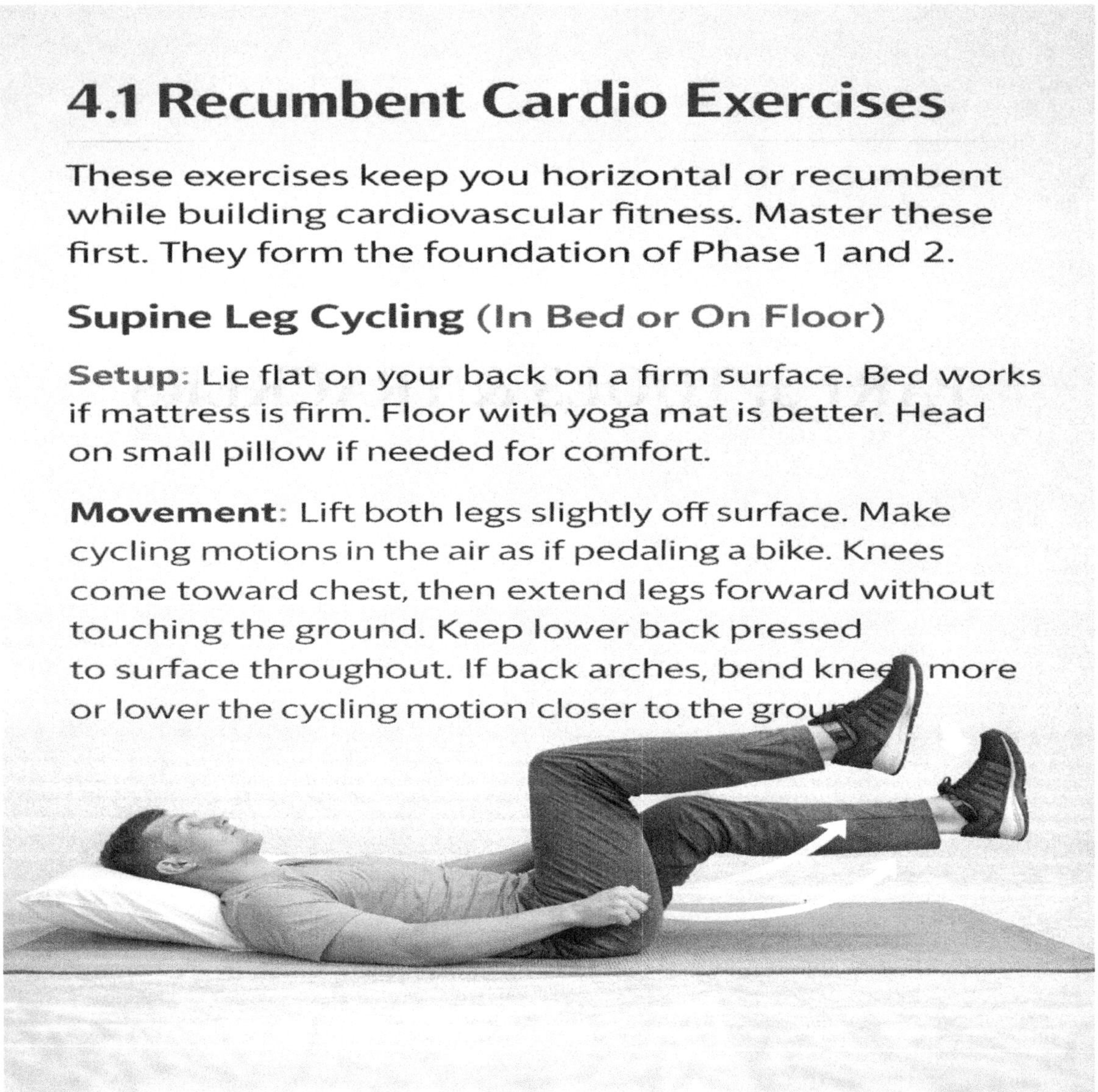

These exercises keep you horizontal or recumbent while building cardiovascular fitness. Master these first. They form the foundation of Phase 1 and 2.

Supine Leg Cycling (In Bed or On Floor)

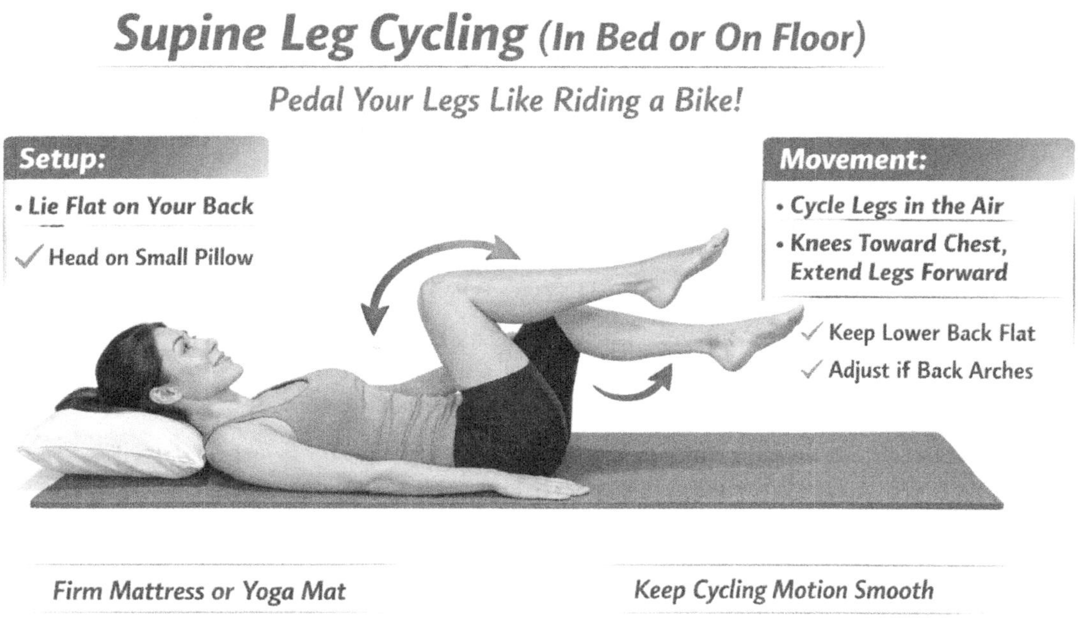
Supine Leg Cycling (In Bed or On Floor)
Pedal Your Legs Like Riding a Bike!
Setup:
• Lie Flat on Your Back
✓ Head on Small Pillow
Movement:
• Cycle Legs in the Air
• Knees Toward Chest, Extend Legs Forward
✓ Keep Lower Back Flat
✓ Adjust if Back Arches
Firm Mattress or Yoga Mat
Keep Cycling Motion Smooth

Setup: Lie flat on your back on a firm surface. Bed works if mattress is firm. Floor with yoga mat is better. Head on small pillow if needed for comfort.

Movement: Lift both legs slightly off surface. Make cycling motions in the air as if pedaling a bike. Knees come toward chest, then extend legs forward without touching the ground. Keep lower back pressed to surface throughout. If back arches, bend knees more or lower the cycling motion closer to the ground.

Breathing: Breathe normally. Don't hold your breath.

Duration: Start with 30-second intervals. Rest 30 seconds. Repeat. Build to 3-5 continuous minutes.

Common mistakes: Arching lower back (fix: bend knees more), holding breath (fix: count out loud), going too fast (fix: slow down, focus on control).

Modifications: Too hard? Keep one foot on ground, cycle with just one leg at a time. Switch legs every 30 seconds. Still too hard? Just march legs in place while lying down, alternating knee lifts.

Recumbent Bike Proper Form

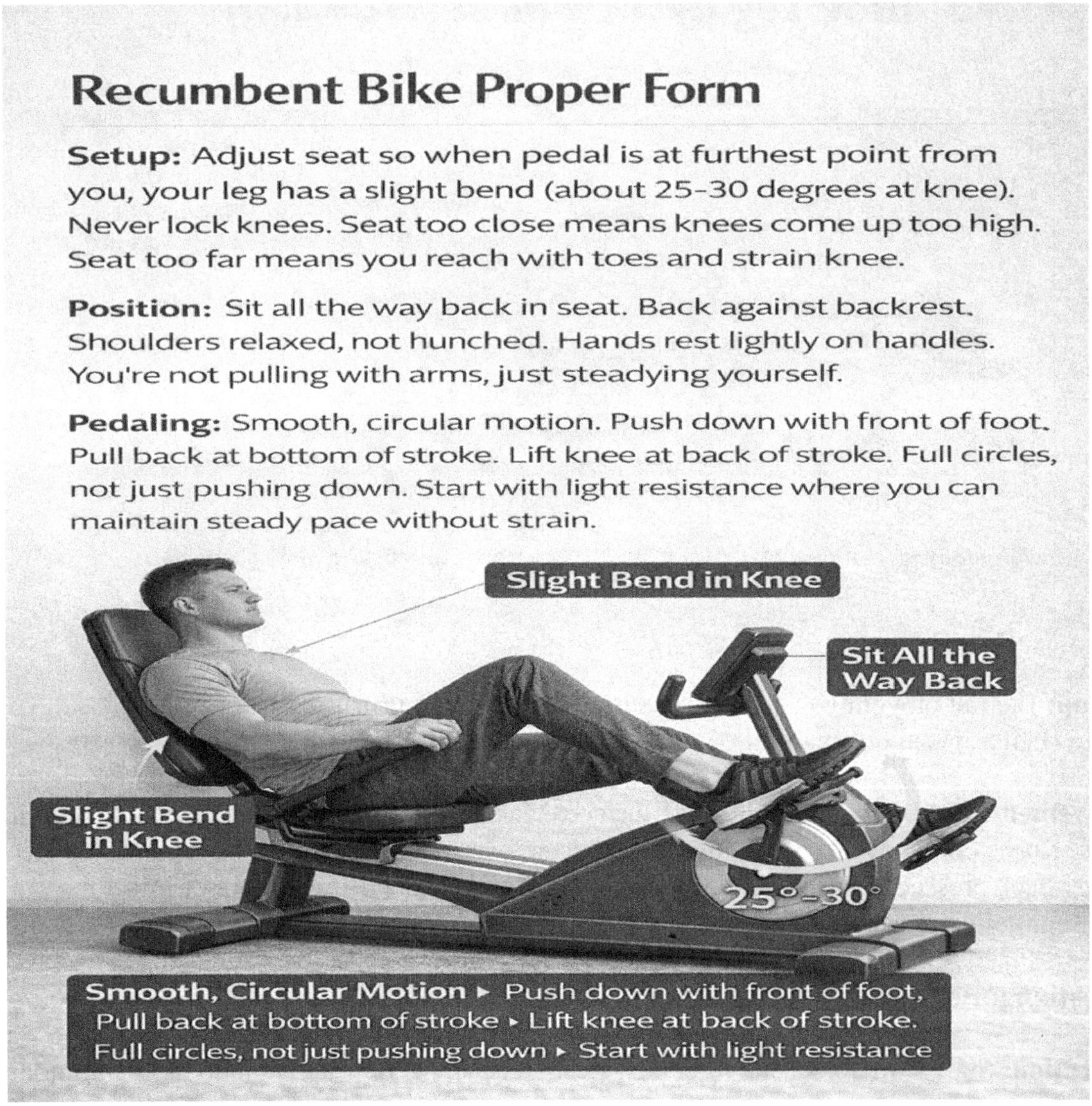

Setup: Adjust seat so when pedal is at furthest point from you, your leg has a slight bend (about 25-30 degrees at knee). Never lock knees. Seat too close means knees come up too high. Seat too far means you reach with toes and strain knee.

Position: Sit all the way back in seat. Back against backrest. Shoulders relaxed, not hunched. Hands rest lightly on handles. You're not pulling with arms, just steadying yourself.

Pedaling: Smooth, circular motion. Push down with front of foot. Pull back at bottom of stroke. Lift knee at back of stroke. Full circles, not just pushing down. Start with light resistance where you can maintain steady pace without strain.

Breathing: Rhythmic breathing matched to pedaling. In for two pedal strokes, out for two pedal strokes.

Heart rate monitoring: Check every 2-3 minutes. Adjust speed or resistance to stay in target zone. If heart rate too high, slow down immediately. Don't wait.

Common mistakes: Seat too close (fix: adjust back one notch), bouncing in seat (fix: lower resistance, pedal smoother), hunched shoulders (fix: relax, sit back), locked knees (fix: adjust seat closer).

Modifications: Knee pain? Check seat height first. Still hurts? Reduce resistance to minimum. Pain continues? Switch to different equipment. Bad knee day? Shorter duration at easier intensity. Don't push through joint pain.

Rowing Machine Technique (Recumbent Position)

Setup: Adjust foot straps so they sit across ball of foot, not toes. Feet secure but not too tight. Sit on seat, knees bent, shins vertical, arms extended holding handle.

The Stroke (Four Parts):

1. **Catch Position:** Knees bent, shins vertical, arms straight, leaning slightly forward from hips.
2. **Drive:** Push with legs first (legs do 60% of work). Legs extend. When legs nearly straight, lean back slightly and pull handle to lower chest. Elbows go past sides.
3. **Finish:** Legs extended (slight bend at knee), leaning back slightly, handle at lower chest.
4. **Recovery:** Extend arms first. Lean forward from hips. Then bend knees, sliding seat forward to catch position.

Rowing Machine Technique

(Recumbent Position)

Setup: Adjust foot straps so they sit across ball of foot, not toes. Feet secure but not too tight. Sit on seat, knees bent, shins vertical, arms extended holding handle.

Movement: Lift both legs slightly off surface. Make cycling motions in the air as if pedaling a bike. Knees come toward chest, then extend legs forward without touching the ground.
Keep lower back pressed to surface throughout.

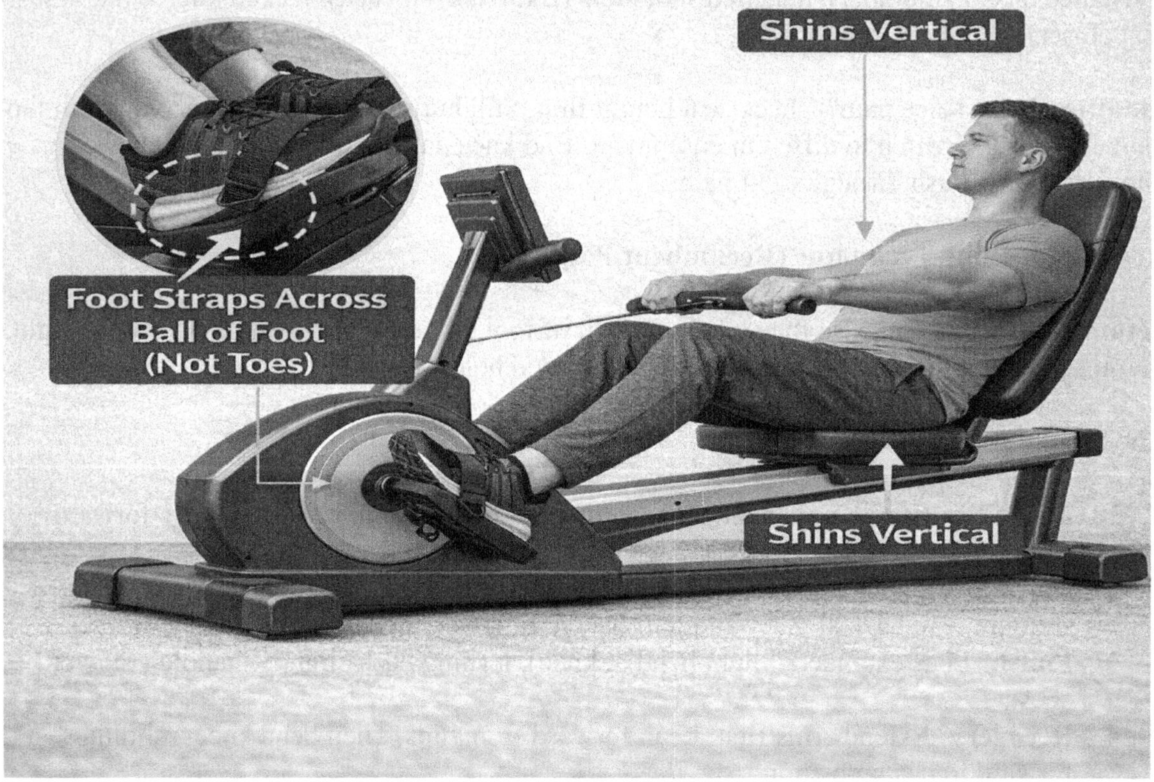

Rhythm: Drive is powerful and quick. Recovery is slow and controlled. Ratio is roughly 1:2. If drive takes 1 second, recovery takes 2 seconds.

Common mistakes: Pulling with arms before legs extend (fix: legs first, always), jerky motion (fix: smooth and controlled), leaning back too far (fix: slight lean only, maintain core), holding breath (fix: exhale on drive, inhale on recovery).

Heart rate note: Rowing works more muscles than bike, so heart rate climbs faster. Monitor closely. Reduce stroke rate if needed, not force.

Modifications: Shoulder problems? Reduce range of motion, don't pull handle all the way to chest. Low back issues? Less lean forward at catch position. Keep torso more upright throughout.

Swimming Modifications

Why swimming works: Water supports body weight. No impact. Stays cool. Pressure from water helps blood return to heart. Excellent for POTS if you have pool access.

Starting position: Float horizontally or vertical with head above water. This is your "recumbent" position in pool.

Movements that work:

- Slow freestyle with frequent rest at wall
- Backstroke (keeps face out of water, easier breathing)
- Water walking in shallow end (upright but water supports body)
- Treading water gently
- Pool noodle or kickboard assisted movements

Guidelines: Start in shallow end where you can stand. Rest at wall frequently. Don't try to swim laps like pre-POTS. This is gentle, sustained movement. Time in water matters more than distance covered.

Heart rate: Harder to check in pool. Use RPE instead. Should feel easy to moderate. If breathing hard, slow down or rest.

Temperature: Cool pool (78-82°F) is better than warm pool for POTS. Warm water can increase symptoms. If pool is too warm, shorter sessions.

Modifications: Can't swim? Use kickboard and just kick. Hold side of pool and walk along edge. Stand in shallow end and march in place. Any movement in water counts.

Chair-Based Cardio Alternatives

For those without equipment or very severe baseline:

Seated Marching:

- Sit in sturdy chair with back support
- Feet flat on floor
- Lift knees alternately as if marching
- Arms can swing naturally
- Start 30 seconds, build to 5 minutes continuous

Seated Jumping Jacks:

- Sit in chair
- Legs: Tap toes wide then together (like jumping jack motion but feet stay on ground)
- Arms: Raise arms overhead then down to sides with leg motion
- Coordination takes practice
- Start 30 seconds, build to 3 minutes

Seated Boxing:

- Sit upright in chair
- Punch alternating arms forward (left, right, left, right)
- Engage core, slight twist with each punch
- Keep shoulders down, don't hunch
- Can add small dumbbells (1-2 lbs) when ready
- Start 1 minute, build to 5 minutes

Seated Step Touch:

- Sit in chair
- Tap right foot to right side, return
- Tap left foot to left side, return
- Arms can swing opposite direction
- Start 1 minute, build to 5 minutes

Progression: Increase duration before increasing intensity. When these feel easy, time to get recumbent bike or pedaler.

4.2 Strength Training Exercises

All strength exercises can be done lying, seated, or standing depending on your program phase. Form matters more than weight or reps. Control beats speed.

Lower Body Exercises

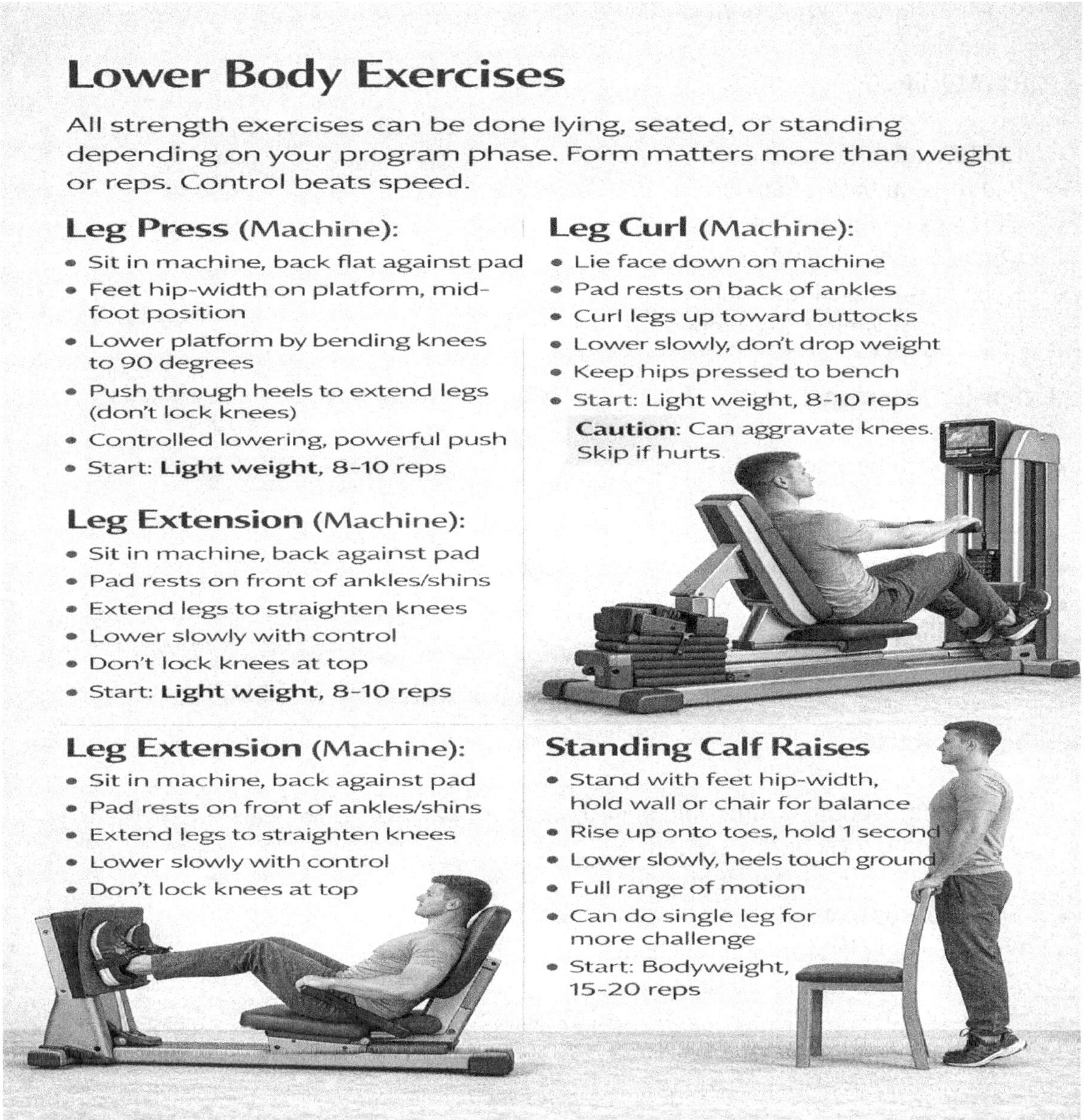

Leg Press (Machine):

- Sit in machine, back flat against pad
- Feet hip-width on platform, mid-foot position
- Lower platform by bending knees to 90 degrees
- Push through heels to extend legs (don't lock knees)
- Controlled lowering, powerful push

- Start: Light weight, 8-10 reps

Leg Curl (Machine):

- Lie face down on machine
- Pad rests on back of ankles
- Curl legs up toward buttocks
- Lower slowly, don't drop weight
- Keep hips pressed to bench
- Start: Light weight, 8-10 reps

Leg Extension (Machine):

- Sit in machine, back against pad
- Pad rests on front of ankles/shins
- Extend legs to straighten knees
- Lower slowly with control
- Don't lock knees at top
- Start: Light weight, 8-10 reps
- Caution: Can aggravate knees. Skip if hurts.

Standing Calf Raises:

- Stand with feet hip-width, hold wall or chair for balance
- Rise up onto toes, hold 1 second
- Lower slowly, heels touch ground
- Full range of motion
- Can do single leg for more challenge
- Start: Bodyweight, 15-20 reps

Core Exercises

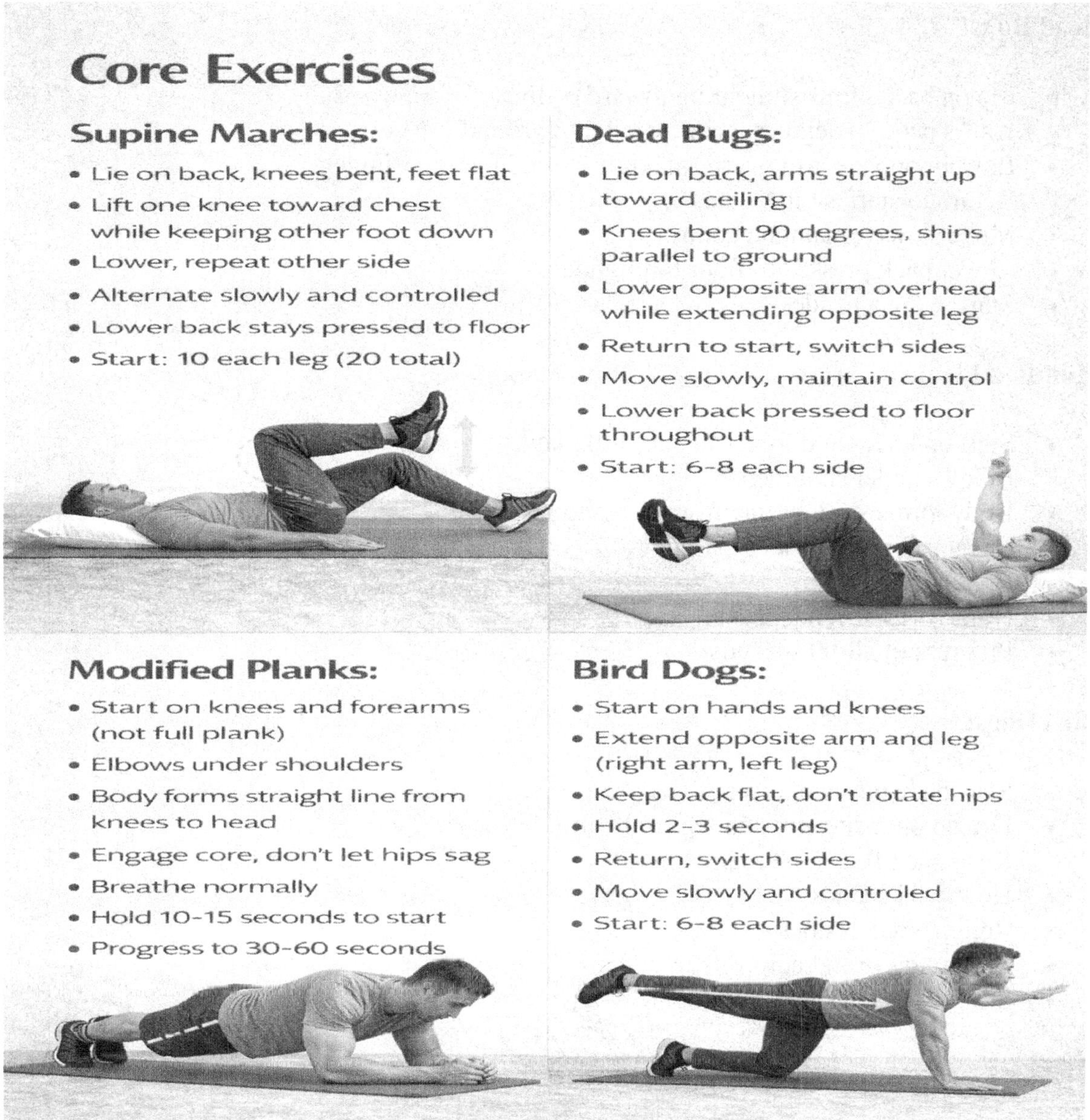

Supine Marches:

- Lie on back, knees bent, feet flat
- Lift one knee toward chest while keeping other foot down
- Lower, repeat other side
- Alternate slowly and controlled
- Lower back stays pressed to floor

- Start: 10 each leg (20 total)

Dead Bugs:

- Lie on back, arms straight up toward ceiling
- Knees bent 90 degrees, shins parallel to ground
- Lower opposite arm overhead while extending opposite leg
- Return to start, switch sides
- Move slowly, maintain control
- Lower back pressed to floor throughout
- Start: 6-8 each side

Modified Planks:

- Start on knees and forearms (not full plank)
- Elbows under shoulders
- Body forms straight line from knees to head
- Engage core, don't let hips sag
- Breathe normally
- Hold 10-15 seconds to start
- Progress to 30-60 seconds

Bird Dogs:

- Start on hands and knees
- Extend opposite arm and leg (right arm, left leg)
- Keep back flat, don't rotate hips
- Hold 2-3 seconds
- Return, switch sides
- Move slowly and controlled
- Start: 6-8 each side

Upper Body Exercises

Upper Body Exercises

Seated Rows (Resistance Band or Cable):

- Sit on floor or bench, legs extended
- Band around feet or attached to stable point
- Pull handles to sides of chest
- Squeeze shoulder blades together
- Extend arms forward slowly.
- Keep back straight, don't round
- Start: 10-12 reps

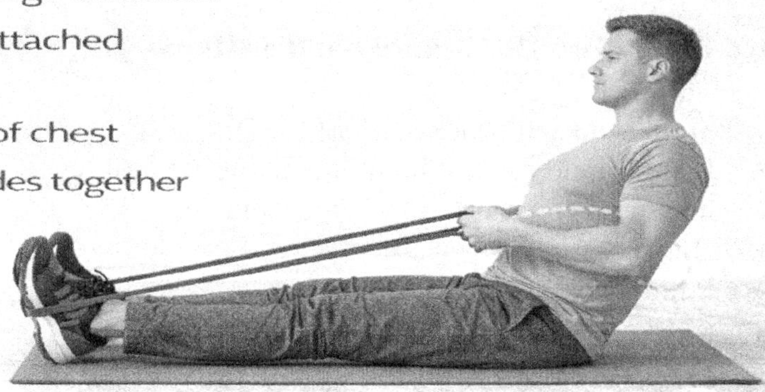

Seated Chest Press (Resistance Band or Dumbbells):

- Sit in chair with back support
- Band behind back or hold dumbbells at chest level
- Press arms forward to full extension
- Don't lock elbows
- Return slowly to start
- Keep core engaged
- Start: 10-12 reps

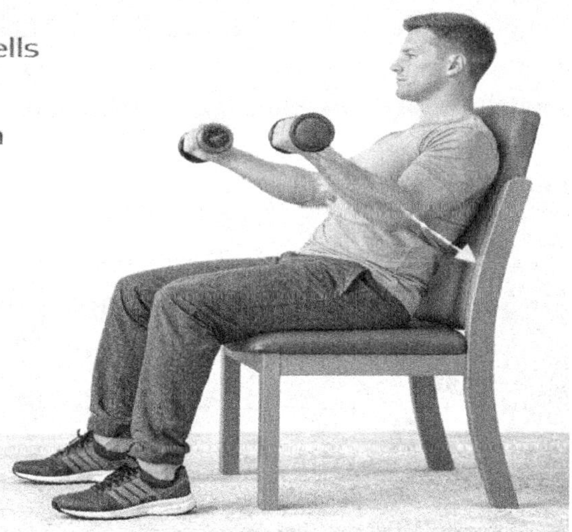

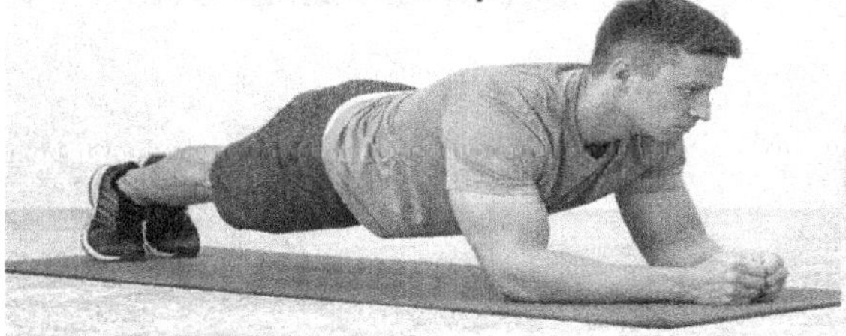

Seated Rows (Resistance Band or Cable):

- Sit on floor or bench, legs extended
- Band around feet or attached to stable point
- Pull handles to sides of chest
- Squeeze shoulder blades together
- Extend arms forward slowly
- Keep back straight, don't round
- Start: 10-12 reps

Seated Chest Press (Resistance Band or Dumbbells):

- Sit in chair with back support
- Band behind back or hold dumbbells at chest level
- Press arms forward to full extension
- Don't lock elbows
- Return slowly to start
- Keep core engaged
- Start: 10-12 reps

Resistance Band Alternatives

Every machine exercise has a band equivalent. Bands are portable, affordable, and effective.

Band Squats: Stand on band, hold handles at shoulders, squat **Band Chest Press:** Anchor behind you, press forward **Band Rows:** Anchor in front, pull to chest **Band Shoulder Press:** Stand on band, press overhead **Band Bicep Curls:** Stand on band, curl up **Band Tricep Extensions:** Hold overhead, extend down

Band Resistance Levels:

- Light (yellow, red): Beginners, high reps
- Medium (green, blue): Intermediate
- Heavy (black, purple): Advanced Start light. Add resistance by shortening band (step wider).

4.3 Upright Cardio Progressions

Use these once you transition to upright exercise in Phase 3 and 4.

Upright Bike Technique

Differences from recumbent:

- You're vertical, fighting gravity
- Heart rate will be 20-30 beats higher for same effort
- More balance required
- Different muscle recruitment

Setup: Seat height so leg has slight bend at bottom of pedal stroke. Handlebars at comfortable height (higher = easier on back). Wear compression garments.

Form: Sit upright, don't hunch forward. Core engaged. Light grip on handlebars. Smooth pedaling motion. Check heart rate every 2-3 minutes.

Progression: Start with 5 minutes upright, increase 2-3 minutes per week. Don't rush this. Upright is significantly harder.

Elliptical Form

Why elliptical: Low impact, natural stride, works whole body, less stress on joints than treadmill.

Setup: Adjust stride length if machine allows. Start with shorter stride. Feet stay flat on pedals throughout.

Form: Stand upright, core engaged. Let machine guide your motion. Push through heels. Don't lean heavily on handles. Light touch for balance only.

Motion: Smooth, gliding movement. No bouncing. If bouncing, resistance is too high or pace too fast.

Heart rate: Climbs quickly on elliptical because whole body works. Monitor closely.

Progression: Start with 5 minutes, slow pace, low resistance. Build time before intensity.

Treadmill Walking (Flat to Incline)

Why walking: Most functional exercise. What you do in daily life. Builds real-world capacity.

Starting flat:

- Speed: 2.0-2.5 mph (slower than normal walking)

- Hands: Light touch on rails initially, progress to hands-free
- Posture: Upright, shoulders back, look forward not down
- Stride: Natural length, full heel-to-toe roll
- Start: 5-10 minutes, progress slowly

Adding incline:

- When: After 2-4 weeks of comfortable flat walking
- Start: 1-2% incline
- Progression: Add 0.5-1% every 1-2 weeks
- Max for POTS: 5-8% (steep inclines spike heart rate dramatically)
- Form: Lean into incline from ankles, not waist. Shorter stride on incline is normal.

Caution: Treadmill requires more balance than bike or elliptical. If dizzy, use bike instead.

Stair Stepping

Real stairs vs machine:

- Real stairs: More functional, free, can control pace
- Machine: Consistent, controlled, easier to monitor heart rate

Technique:

- Full foot on each step, not just toes
- Push through heel
- Use railing lightly for balance
- Upright posture
- Controlled pace, no rushing

Progression:

- Start: 1 flight, rest, repeat 2-3 times
- Progress: Add flights or reduce rest
- Descending: Go slow, easier on heart than ascending

When to use: Late Phase 3 or Phase 4 once upright tolerance solid. Stairs are intense.

Exercise 4.3A: Equipment Inventory

List what you have access to and what you'll use for the program.

Recumbent cardio options I have:

[ ] Recumbent bike [ ] Supine pedaler [ ] Rowing machine [ ] Pool [ ] Chair-based only

Upright cardio options I have:

[ ] Upright bike [ ] Elliptical [ ] Treadmill [ ] Real stairs [ ] None yet

Strength training equipment I have:

[ ] Resistance bands [ ] Dumbbells [ ] Gym access [ ] Bodyweight only

Equipment I need to acquire:

1. ______________________________
2. ______________________________
3. ______________________________

Where I'll exercise:

Home:

____

Gym:

____

Other:

____

Backup plan if primary equipment unavailable:

____

____

4.4 Form Checks

Exercise 4.4A: Practice and Self-Assess

Choose one cardio and two strength exercises. Practice them. Check your form.

Cardio exercise I practiced: ______________________________

What I did correctly:

____

____

What I need to improve:

____

____

Strength exercise 1 I practiced: ______________________________

Form points I focused on:

____

____

Strength exercise 2 I practiced: ______________________________

Form points I focused on:

____

____

Questions I still have about form:

____

____

____

4.5 Quick Reference

- Form beats speed or weight every time
- Check heart rate frequently when learning new exercises
- Pain means stop, reassess, modify
- Breathe throughout all exercises, never hold breath
- Modify rather than skip when exercise too hard
- Master recumbent before attempting upright
- Use this chapter as reference throughout program

Chapter 5.0: Your Tracking System

Tracking is how you see progress when symptoms lie to you. You'll feel like nothing is changing. The data will prove otherwise. This chapter gives you every tracking tool needed for 16 weeks. Use them consistently. They become your proof that the protocol works.

5.1 Why Track

Your subjective experience is unreliable. On hard days, you'll feel like you're failing. On good days, you'll forget how bad things were. Data doesn't lie. You need objective evidence of progress. Three months from now, you'll look back at Week 1 logs and barely recognize that person. That's what tracking gives you.

What you'll track:

- Exercise duration, intensity, heart rate
- How you feel during and after exercise
- Symptoms day-to-day
- Standing tolerance
- Monthly progress comparisons

How to use the data:

- Identify patterns (best time of day, equipment, etc.)
- Catch problems early (overtraining, inadequate recovery)
- Prove progress when you can't feel it
- Share with doctor at checkups
- Motivate yourself when discouraged

5.2 Daily Exercise Logs

Use these after every cardio session. Takes 2 minutes. Do it immediately post-exercise while memory fresh.

Daily Exercise Log Template

Date: __________ **Week:** _____ **Day:** _____

Cardio Session:

Equipment used:

____

Planned duration: _____ min Actual duration: _____ min

Position: [ ] Recumbent [ ] Upright [ ] Mixed

Target HR zone: _____% Actual HR: Start _____ Mid _____ End _____ Peak _____

RPE (1-10): _____

How I felt during exercise (1-10, where 10=great): _____

Symptoms during exercise: (check all that apply)

[ ] None [ ] Lightheaded [ ] Dizzy [ ] Nausea [ ] Heart racing [ ] Chest tightness [ ] Shortness of breath [ ] Extreme fatigue [ ] Shaky [ ] Brain fog [ ] Other:

____

How I felt 2-4 hours after (1-10): _____

How I felt next morning (1-10): _____

Strength Training: [ ] Completed [ ] Skipped

Exercises done:

____

Notes on today's session:

____

____

____

Exercise 5.2A: Set Up Your System

Decide how you'll track. Choose one method and commit to it.

My tracking method: (check one)

[ ] Paper logs (print or write in this workbook) [ ] Spreadsheet (Excel, Google Sheets) [ ] App (specify: ____) [ ]

Notebook dedicated to tracking [ ] Other:

____

Where I'll keep my tracking tools:

____

When I'll complete daily logs: (right after exercise, before bed, etc.)

____

Who will help hold me accountable to tracking:

____

5.3 Weekly Summary Sheets

Complete these every Sunday evening. Review the week. Look for patterns. Plan improvements.

Week _____ Summary (Dates: __________ to __________)

Cardio sessions completed: _____ out of _____ planned

Total cardio minutes this week: _____ minutes

Strength sessions completed: _____ out of _____ planned

Sessions missed: _____

Reasons:

____

____

Average intensity:

[ ] Easier than prescribed [ ] On target [ ] Harder than prescribed

Average "feeling" during exercise: _____ (out of 10)

Average "feeling" 2-4 hours after: _____ (out of 10)

Most common symptoms this week:

Best session of the week: (day, why it went well)

Hardest session of the week: (day, what made it difficult)

What I learned this week:

What I'll adjust for next week:

Sleep average: _____ hours per night

Hydration: [ ] Excellent [ ] Good [ ] Needs improvement

Sodium intake: [ ] Met goal [ ] Close [ ] Too low

Overall week rating (1-10): _____

5.4 Monthly Progress Reviews

Complete these at the end of Weeks 4, 8, 12, and 16. Big picture assessment.

Month _____ Progress Review (End of Week _____)

Total cardio sessions this month: _____ out of _____ possible

Completion rate: _____%

Total exercise minutes this month: _____ minutes

Average session duration: _____ minutes

Longest single session: _____ minutes (Week _____)

Measurements:

Resting HR lying: _____ Baseline: _____ Change: _____

Standing HR 1 min: _____ Baseline: _____ Change: _____

Standing HR 3 min: _____ Baseline: _____ Change: _____

Standing tolerance: _____ min Baseline: _____ Change: _____

Symptom changes this month:

Better:

____

____

Worse:

____

____

Unchanged:

____

____

Physical changes noticed:

____

____

____

Activities I can do now that I couldn't do at month start:

Biggest accomplishment this month:

Biggest challenge this month:

Looking ahead to next month:

My goal: ______________________________

One thing I'll focus on: ______________________________

5.5 Standing Tolerance Log

Track this weekly. Simple test: how long can you stand still before symptoms force you to sit?

Instructions: Stand still in one place (kitchen, bathroom, etc.). No walking, no leaning. Hands at sides or lightly touching counter for balance only. Start timer. Stand until you must sit due to symptoms. Record time and symptoms that ended the test.

Week _____ Standing Test

Date: __________ Time of day: __________

Standing duration: _____ minutes _____ seconds

Symptoms that ended test: ______________________________

How quickly symptoms resolved after sitting: ____

Exercise 5.5A: Baseline Standing Test

Do this before starting the program. Repeat monthly.

Baseline Standing Test

Date: __________ Time: __________

Duration: _____ min _____ sec

Symptoms:
____

Week 4 Retest

Date: __________ Time: __________

Duration: _____ min _____ sec Change from baseline: _____

Symptoms:
____

Week 8 Retest

Date: __________ Time: __________

Duration: _____ min _____ sec Change from baseline: _____

Symptoms:
____

Week 12 Retest

Date: __________ Time: __________

Duration: _____ min _____ sec Change from baseline: _____

Symptoms:

____

Week 16 Retest

Date: __________ Time: __________

Duration: _____ min _____ sec Change from baseline: _____

Symptoms:

____

5.6 Photo Progress Option

Numbers tell one story. Photos tell another. Optional but powerful.

Take photos at baseline, Week 4, Week 8, Week 12, and Week 16. Same clothing, same location, same time of day, same lighting.

Photo guidelines:

- Front view, side view
- Wear fitted clothing or athletic wear
- Same outfit for all progress photos
- Neutral expression
- Store privately for your eyes only
- Compare at end of program

Not about weight or appearance. About posture changes. Muscle definition. How you carry yourself. Confidence that shows in stance.

5.7 Organizing Your Data

Exercise 5.7A: Create Your Tracking Routine

Plan exactly how you'll stay organized for 16 weeks.

My daily tracking routine:

After each exercise session, I will: ____

____

Time required: _____ minutes

My weekly tracking routine:

Every Sunday, I will: ____

____

Time required: _____ minutes

My monthly tracking routine:

End of Weeks 4, 8, 12, 16, I will: ____

____

Time required: _____ minutes

Where I'll store all tracking materials:

____

Digital backup plan: (if using paper)

____

What I'll do if I miss logging a day:

____

____

5.8 Quick Reference

- Track every session, no exceptions
- Log immediately after exercise
- Weekly reviews every Sunday
- Monthly reviews at end of Weeks 4, 8, 12, 16
- Standing tolerance tests monthly
- Data reveals patterns you can't feel
- Three months of data = undeniable proof of progress

Chapter 6.0: Troubleshooting and Modifications

Things will go wrong. You'll crash. You'll get sick. You'll have terrible days. This chapter is your emergency manual. Refer to it when problems arise. Keep the protocol going even when perfect execution isn't possible.

6.1 I Crashed Now What

You crashed. You did everything right and still crashed. Or you pushed too hard and crashed. Either way, you're here now. Here's the protocol.

Immediate actions:

1. Complete rest for 24-48 hours (no structured exercise)
2. Increase sodium and fluid intake
3. Stay horizontal as much as possible
4. Sleep as much as your body wants
5. Don't panic (this happens, it's recoverable)

Determining crash severity:

Mild crash: Symptoms 20-30% worse than baseline, can still function, resolves in 1-2 days **Action:** Take 1-2 days off, resume at previous week's prescription

Moderate crash: Symptoms 50%+ worse, struggle with basic activities, resolves in 3-5 days **Action:** Take 3-4 days off, drop back one full week when resuming, rebuild slowly

Severe crash: Symptoms back to pre-program baseline or worse, bedridden, takes week+ to resolve **Action:** Take full week off minimum, drop back to Week 1 when resuming, investigate cause thoroughly

When to resume exercise after crash:

- Symptoms back to baseline
- Two consecutive good days
- Adequate sleep (8+ hours)
- Not fighting illness
- Mentally ready to start again

How to resume:

- Start at lower intensity than where you crashed
- Reduce duration by 25-50%
- Add one variable at a time (time, then intensity)
- Track meticulously to catch early warning signs
- Takes 1-2 weeks to get back to pre-crash level

Exercise 6.1A: Crash Protocol Checklist

Complete this if you crash. Helps identify cause and plan recovery.

Date of crash: __________

Crash severity: [ ] Mild [ ] Moderate [ ] Severe

Symptoms: (check all that apply)

[ ] Extreme fatigue [ ] Can't get out of bed [ ] Severe lightheadedness [ ] Nausea [ ] Heart racing at rest [ ] Chest pain [ ] Severe headache [ ] Cognitive impairment [ ] Flu-like symptoms [ ] Other: ____

What I was doing when crash hit:

____

____

Possible causes: (check all that apply)

[ ] Pushed too hard in exercise [ ] Increased intensity too fast [ ] Inadequate recovery [ ] Poor sleep previous night [ ] Illness brewing [ ] Inadequate sodium/hydration [ ] Exercised during POTS flare [ ] Hot weather [ ] Hormonal changes [ ] Stress [ ] Other:

____

My recovery plan:

Days off: _____

When I'll resume: __________

How I'll modify:

____

How I'll prevent this in future:**

6.2 Regression Strategies

Sometimes you need to take two steps back to take three steps forward. That's not failure. That's strategy.

When to regress:

- Three consecutive sessions feel much harder than they should
- Symptoms increasing despite following protocol
- Sleep quality declining
- Resting heart rate elevated by 10+ beats
- Dread or anxiety about exercise sessions
- Post-exercise crashes becoming frequent

How to regress effectively:

Option 1: Drop duration

- Reduce duration by 25-50%
- Keep intensity same
- Stay at reduced duration until feeling solid (3-5 sessions)
- Build back up slowly

Option 2: Drop intensity

- Keep duration same
- Drop down one heart rate zone
- Stay there until recovery improves
- Gradually increase intensity again

Option 3: Drop frequency

- Reduce from 6 days to 4-5 days per week

- Extra rest days for recovery
- Maintain quality over quantity
- Add days back when ready

Option 4: Repeat previous week

- Literally redo the previous week's prescription
- Master it before advancing
- No shame in repeating weeks

Regression is not quitting: You're recalibrating. The protocol is a guide, not a law. Your body determines the pace.

Exercise 6.2A: Design Your Regression

If you need to regress, use this template to plan it.

Current prescription I'm struggling with:

Week: _____ Duration: _____ Intensity: _____ Frequency: _____ days/week

What specifically feels too hard:

____

____

My regression plan: (choose one or combine)

[ ] Reduce duration to: _____ minutes

[ ] Reduce intensity to: __________ zone or RPE ______

[ ] Reduce frequency to: _____ days per week

[ ] Repeat Week: _____

How long I'll stay at regression level: _____ sessions or _____ weeks

Signs I'm ready to progress again:

____

____

6.3 Managing Heat Intolerance

Heat makes POTS worse. Summer is brutal. Here's how to keep exercising when it's hot.

Why heat matters: Heat causes blood vessels to dilate. Blood pools more. Heart works harder. Symptoms spike. Dehydration accelerates.

Solutions:

Cool environment:

- Exercise in air conditioning (ideal)
- Use fan directly on you
- Morning exercise before heat builds
- Evening after sun down
- Avoid midday heat

Body cooling:

- Ice pack on neck during exercise
- Cooling vest if accessible
- Cold wet towel on head and neck
- Cold shower before exercise
- Cold drink during and after

Hydration:

- Increase fluid intake by 50%
- Add electrolyte drinks
- Drink cold fluids (helps core temp)
- Pre-load 16-20 oz before exercise
- Continue drinking during

Modifications:

- Reduce intensity one zone
- Shorten duration by 25%
- Extra recovery days
- Switch to pool if available (best option)

When to skip: Temperature over 85°F without AC, humidity over 70%, or you're already overheated from daily activities. Don't force it. Live to exercise another day.

6.4 Period and Menstrual Cycle

Hormones affect POTS symptoms. Periods make everything harder. Plan for it.

Typical pattern:

- Week before period: Symptoms worsen
- First 2-3 days of period: Worst symptoms
- Days 3-7 of period: Gradual improvement
- Week after period: Often best week of month

Modifications during period:

Days 1-3 (worst):

- Drop intensity one zone
- Reduce duration by 25-50%
- Extra rest day if needed
- Focus on completing something, anything
- Don't expect PRs

Days 4-7 (improving):

- Gradually return to normal prescription
- Listen to body day by day
- Resume full program when bleeding light or stopped

Premenstrual week:

- Expect symptoms to worsen
- May need slight modifications
- Increase sodium and hydration
- Plan lighter week in advance

Post-menstrual week:

- Often best week for progression
- Take advantage of good symptom window
- Push slightly harder if feeling strong

What doesn't work: Forcing full prescription on worst period days. You'll crash. Better to modify proactively than recover from crash.

Exercise 6.4A: Track Your Cycle

Monitor exercise tolerance across your cycle. Patterns will emerge.

My typical cycle length: _____ days

Period duration: _____ days

Days I feel worst: (mark on calendar)

Day 1-3 of period: [ ] Day 4-7 of period: [ ] Week before period: [ ] Other: ______

My period modification plan:

Days 1-3:

____

____

Days 4-7:

____

____

Week before:

____

____

6.5 Illness or Infection Rules

When you're sick, the rules change. Here's the protocol.

General guideline: Symptoms above the neck vs. below the neck.

Above neck (runny nose, sore throat, head cold, sinus congestion):

- Light exercise okay if you feel okay
- Drop intensity significantly (Recovery zone only)
- Shorten duration by 50%
- Listen to body each day
- Stop if you feel worse mid-session

Below neck (chest congestion, cough, body aches, fever, stomach issues):

- Complete rest until resolved
- No exercise with fever ever
- No exercise with chest infection
- Wait until symptoms gone plus one good day
- Resume at previous week's prescription

COVID-19 or flu:

- Complete rest until symptoms resolved
- Add 7 days post-symptom resolution before exercising
- Resume at Week 1 prescription
- Rebuild slowly over 2-4 weeks
- Watch for post-viral POTS worsening

When in doubt: Rest. One missed week better than four weeks recovering from pushing through illness.

6.6 Equipment Free Alternatives

No equipment? No problem. Here are substitutions.

Recumbent cardio without equipment:

- Supine leg cycling in bed (described in Chapter 4.0)
- Supine marching in bed
- Chair cardio (seated marching, seated jacks)

Upright cardio without equipment:

- Walking outside or in house
- Marching in place
- Step touch side to side
- Stair climbing in home

Strength without equipment:

- Bodyweight exercises (squats, lunges, push-ups from knees)
- Wall sits
- Calf raises holding counter
- Planks and side planks

- Glute bridges and single-leg bridges
- Resistance from household items (water bottles, canned goods)

Makeshift equipment:

- Backpack with books = weight vest
- Towel = resistance band
- Stairs = cardio and strength
- Wall = support for balance exercises
- Chair = bench for step-ups

Exercise 6.6A: Plan Equipment Free Workouts

Design three workouts using zero equipment.

Workout 1 (Recumbent Cardio):

Exercises:

____

____

Duration: _____ minutes

Workout 2 (Upright Cardio):

Exercises:

____

____

Duration: _____ minutes

Workout 3 (Strength):

Exercises:

____

____

____

Duration: _____ minutes

6.7 Seated Only for Severe Cases

If you can't do recumbent yet, start seated. Work to recumbent, then to upright.

Seated progression:

- Week 1-2: Chair cardio 3-5 minutes
- Week 3-4: Chair cardio 5-10 minutes
- Week 5-6: Transition to supine cycling in bed 5-10 minutes
- Week 7-8: Continue supine work, build to 15-20 minutes
- Week 9+: Begin recumbent bike or pedaler if symptoms allow

Seated strength:

- All exercises done from chair
- Focus on upper body first (less orthostatic stress)
- Add lower body as tolerated
- Resistance bands attach to chair legs

When to progress: Two consecutive weeks of completing prescribed work without symptom increase.

6.8 Working Around Comorbidities

EDS (Ehlers-Danlos Syndrome) modifications:

- Never lock joints
- Focus on stability over flexibility
- Lower resistance, higher control
- Avoid hyperextension
- Support vulnerable joints
- May need physical therapist guidance for form

MCAS (Mast Cell Activation Syndrome) modifications:

- Avoid overheating (major trigger)
- Pre-exercise antihistamines
- Cool environment essential
- Watch for flushing, hives, breathing issues
- Have emergency medications accessible
- May need to exercise in shorter bouts

ME/CFS (Myalgic Encephalomyelitis) modifications:

- Risk of post-exertional malaise (PEM)
- Start extremely conservative (2-3 minutes)
- Increase very slowly (30 seconds per week)
- May need longer rest between sessions
- Pay close attention to delayed crashes (24-72 hours post)
- Consult ME/CFS specialist about exercise safety

Exercise 6.8A: My Comorbidity Plan

If you have comorbidities, detail your modifications.

My comorbidities:

____

____

Specific modifications I need:

____

____

____

____

Warning signs to watch for:

____

____

When to stop immediately:

____

____

6.9 Quick Reference

- Crashes happen, they're recoverable
- Regress when needed, progress when ready
- Modify for heat, periods, illness
- Equipment free options exist
- Comorbidities require specific modifications

- Better to modify than to crash
- Consistency beats perfection

Chapter 7.0: Beyond Week 16

You finished 16 weeks. You reconditioned your cardiovascular system. Now what? This chapter is about maintaining gains, continuing progress, and living life beyond the structured protocol.

7.1 Transition to Self Directed

The training wheels come off. You've learned how your body responds to exercise. Now you apply that knowledge independently.

What you know now:

- Your ideal heart rate zones
- Best time of day for exercise
- How much recovery you need
- Early warning signs of overdoing it
- Equipment you prefer
- Your symptom patterns

Shifting mindset: From "following protocol" to "maintaining fitness." From "building capacity" to "using capacity." You're not done exercising. You're done with the structured 16-week build. Now you maintain.

Maintenance requirements:

- 3-5 exercise sessions per week (down from 5-6)
- 30-45 minutes per session
- Mix of intensities (mostly Base Pace and Maximal Steady State)
- 1-2 strength sessions per week
- Listen to body, not rigid schedule

Exercise 7.1A: Design Your Maintenance Plan

Create a realistic weekly schedule you'll actually follow.

Days I'll exercise: (check all that apply)

[ ] Monday [ ] Tuesday [ ] Wednesday [ ] Thursday [ ] Friday [ ] Saturday [ ] Sunday

Typical week structure:

Monday:

____

Tuesday:

____

Wednesday:

____

Thursday:

____

Friday:

____

Saturday:

____

Sunday:

____

Duration per session: _____ minutes

Mix of activities I'll do:

____

____

____

How I'll track maintenance: (still track, just less detailed)

____

____

7.2 Keeping Progressive Safely

Maintenance doesn't mean stagnation. You can still improve. Just more slowly and carefully.

Safe progression options:

Option 1: Increase duration

- Add 5 minutes per session every 2-4 weeks
- Max out at 60 minutes for POTS (longer doesn't necessarily help more)

Option 2: Increase intensity

- Spend more time at Maximal Steady State
- Add interval sessions 1-2x per week
- Experiment with brief intervals at 80-85% max HR

Option 3: Increase variety

- Try new activities (hiking, cycling outdoors, dance classes, sports)
- Add challenge in different ways (terrain, weather, group settings)

Option 4: Increase strength

- Progress resistance training (heavier weights, more sets)
- Add advanced exercises (single leg work, unstable surfaces)

Choose one progression at a time. Don't increase duration and intensity simultaneously. One variable per month maximum.

When to stop progressing: When current fitness level allows you to do everything you want to do in life. Fitness is a tool for living, not an end itself.

Exercise 7.2A: My Six Month Goals

Set realistic goals for the next six months post-program.

By 6 months post-program, I want to:

Physical goal:

____

____

Activity goal:

____

____

Functional goal: ____

____

To achieve these, I'll:

____

____

____

How I'll know I've succeeded:

____

____

7.3 Returning to Favorite Activities

You've rebuilt capacity. Time to use it. Return to activities you couldn't do before.

Activities to try:

- Walking distances that were impossible pre-program
- Shopping without wheelchair or frequent sitting
- Playing with kids or pets
- Hiking easy trails
- Dancing at events
- Standing at concerts or gatherings
- Light recreational sports
- Gardening for extended periods
- Traveling with less symptom management

Reintroduction strategy:

- Start shorter/easier than you think you should
- Build up gradually over weeks
- Don't abandon exercise maintenance to add activities
- Activities supplement exercise, don't replace it

Managing expectations: You've improved significantly. You're not cured. You still have POTS. Choose activities that match your new capacity, not your pre-POTS capacity.

Exercise 7.3A: Activity Bucket List

List activities you want to try now that you've reconditioned.

Activities I couldn't do before but want to try now:

1. ______________________________
2. ______________________________
3. ______________________________
4. ______________________________
5. ______________________________

Activity I'll try first: ______________________________

When I'll try it: __________

How I'll prepare:

____

____

Modifications I might need:

____

____

7.4 Fitness Maintenance Schedules

Different maintenance schedules for different lifestyles.

Minimal Maintenance (3 days/week):

- Monday: 30 min cardio, strength
- Wednesday: 30 min cardio
- Saturday: 40-45 min cardio, strength
- Maintains current fitness, won't progress much
- Good for busy periods

Standard Maintenance (4 days/week):

- Monday: 35 min cardio
- Tuesday: Strength training

- Thursday: 35 min cardio with intervals
- Saturday: 40 min cardio, strength
- Maintains with room for slight progression
- Balanced for most people

Active Maintenance (5 days/week):

- Monday: 40 min cardio
- Tuesday: Strength
- Wednesday: 30 min cardio
- Thursday: Strength
- Saturday: 45 min cardio
- Allows continued progression
- For those who enjoy exercise and have time

Choose based on: Your schedule, energy levels, goals, enjoyment of exercise.

7.5 Recognizing Deconditioning

Your fitness isn't permanent. Skip exercise for weeks, you'll lose gains. Watch for these signs.

Early warning signs:

- Exercise feels harder than it did
- Heart rate higher for same effort
- Recovery takes longer
- Standing tolerance decreasing
- Symptoms creeping back
- Resting heart rate increasing

If caught early: Resume regular exercise, gains return quickly (1-2 weeks).

If ignored: May need to repeat portions of protocol.

Prevention:

- Exercise minimum 3x per week
- Don't skip more than one week
- Track periodically (once per month minimum)
- Retest standing tolerance quarterly
- Stay aware of symptom trends

Exercise 7.5A: Create Your Deconditioning Alarm

Define specific markers that will alert you to slipping backwards.

My deconditioning warning signs:

Resting HR increase: If resting HR goes above _____, I'm deconditioning

Standing tolerance: If I can't stand for _____ minutes, I'm backsliding

Exercise HR: If HR at usual pace exceeds _____, something's wrong

Subjective: If exercise feels significantly harder for _____ consecutive sessions

Symptoms: If these symptoms return:
____

____

What I'll do if I notice deconditioning:

Step 1:
____

Step 2:
____

Step 3:
____

7.6 When to Repeat Protocol

Sometimes life happens. You get sick. You stop exercising. You decondition significantly. When do you repeat the full 16 weeks?

Repeat full protocol if:

- Stopped exercising for 3+ months
- Major illness caused significant deconditioning
- Pregnancy and postpartum period
- Surgery or extended medical recovery
- Symptoms return to pre-program baseline

- Standing tolerance back to starting point

Don't need full repeat if:

- Stopped for 2-6 weeks only
- Can jump back in at Week 8-10 level
- Resume maintenance, rebuild over 3-4 weeks

Modified repeat: Start at Week 5-6, progress through to Week 16. Skips the very basic foundation since you've done it before. Takes 12 weeks instead of 16.

Exercise 7.6A: My Restart Plan

Plan now for potential future deconditioning.

If I decondition and need to restart, I'll:

____

____

Support I'll need to restart:

____

____

How I'll motivate myself to start again:

____

____

____

Reminder to future me:

____

____

____

____

7.7 Long Term Sustainability

Exercise is now part of your POTS management. Like medication, sodium, fluids, compression. It's not optional.

Making it sustainable:

- Find activities you enjoy (if you hate it, you'll quit)
- Exercise with others when possible (accountability and social)
- Vary activities to prevent boredom
- Set new goals periodically (races, hikes, trips)
- Track just enough to stay accountable (not obsessively)
- Give yourself grace on hard days
- Remember why you started

Integration with life:

- Schedule exercise like appointments
- Prepare gym bag night before
- Remove barriers (equipment at home, gym near work)
- Link to existing habits (exercise after coffee, before dinner)
- Make it non-negotiable (like brushing teeth)

When exercise gets hard again: Remember Week 1. Remember not being able to do 3 minutes. Remember how far you've come. Use that as fuel.

7.8 Final Words

You did something most POTS patients never attempt. You reconditioned your cardiovascular system through 16 weeks of consistent work. Your heart is larger. Your blood volume is higher. Your symptoms are better. This is your achievement.

Exercise didn't cure your POTS. It gave you more life within your POTS. That's worth maintaining. Keep moving. Keep tracking. Keep showing up. Your body can do more than you thought possible. You proved that. Don't forget it.

7.9 Quick Reference

- Maintain with 3-5 sessions per week
- Progress slowly and carefully if desired
- Return to favorite activities gradually
- Watch for signs of deconditioning
- Repeat protocol if needed after long breaks
- Track periodically to stay accountable
- Exercise is now part of POTS management forever
- You've got this

APPENDICES

Appendix A: Heart Rate Zone Calculators

Use these worksheets to calculate your personalized heart rate zones. You'll reference these throughout the entire 16-week program. Complete this before starting Week 1.

A.1 Standard Heart Rate Calculation

For those NOT on beta blockers or medications that affect heart rate

Step 1: Calculate Maximum Heart Rate

Maximum Heart Rate = 220 - Age

My age: _____ years

220 - _____ = _____ beats per minute (bpm)

My Maximum Heart Rate: _____ bpm

Step 2: Calculate Each Training Zone

Recovery Zone (50-60% of max HR)

Lower end: _____ (max HR) × 0.50 = _____ bpm

Upper end: _____ (max HR) × 0.60 = _____ bpm

My Recovery Zone: _____ to _____ bpm

Base Pace Zone (60-70% of max HR)

Lower end: _____ (max HR) × 0.60 = _____ bpm

Upper end: _____ (max HR) × 0.70 = _____ bpm

My Base Pace Zone: _____ to _____ bpm

Maximal Steady State Zone (70-80% of max HR)

Lower end: _____ (max HR) × 0.70 = _____ bpm

Upper end: _____ (max HR) × 0.80 = _____ bpm

My Maximal Steady State Zone: _____ to _____ bpm

Interval Training Zone (80-90% of max HR)

Lower end: _____ (max HR) × 0.80 = _____ bpm

Upper end: _____ (max HR) × 0.90 = _____ bpm

My Interval Training Zone: _____ to _____ bpm

Example Calculation (Age 28):

- Max HR: 220 - 28 = 192 bpm
- Recovery: 192 × 0.50 = 96 bpm to 192 × 0.60 = 115 bpm
- Base Pace: 192 × 0.60 = 115 bpm to 192 × 0.70 = 134 bpm
- Maximal Steady State: 192 × 0.70 = 134 bpm to 192 × 0.80 = 154 bpm
- Interval: 192 × 0.80 = 154 bpm to 192 × 0.90 = 173 bpm

A.2 RPE Scale for Beta Blocker Users

For those on beta blockers or heart rate-limiting medications

Beta blockers prevent your heart rate from increasing normally during exercise. Use Rate of Perceived Exertion (RPE) instead of heart rate zones.

RPE Scale (1-10):

1-2: Very Easy - Can talk easily, barely feel like exercising **3-4: Easy (Recovery Zone)** - Can hold conversation, breathing slightly elevated **5-6: Moderate (Base Pace)** - Can talk in short sentences, working but sustainable **7-8: Hard (Maximal Steady State)** - Can only speak a few words, breathing hard **9-10: Very Hard (Intervals)** - Cannot talk, maximum effort

My RPE to Heart Rate Zone Conversion:

Recovery Zone = RPE 3-4 Base Pace Zone = RPE 5-6 Maximal Steady State = RPE 7-8 Interval Training = RPE 9-10

Medications I take that affect heart rate:

I will use: [ ] Heart rate zones [ ] RPE scale [ ] Both (comparing)

A.3 Quick Reference Card

Copy this and keep with your exercise equipment:

```
MY HEART RATE ZONES

Age: _____ Max HR: _____ bpm

Recovery: _____ to _____ bpm (RPE 3-4)
Base Pace: _____ to _____ bpm (RPE 5-6)
Maximal Steady State: _____ to _____ bpm (RPE 7-8)
Interval: _____ to _____ bpm (RPE 9-10)

Phase 1 (Weeks 1-4): Recovery to Base Pace
Phase 2 (Weeks 5-8): Base Pace to Maximal Steady State
Phase 3 (Weeks 9-12): Base Pace to Maximal Steady State (introducing upright)
Phase 4 (Weeks 13-16): Full range including intervals
```

A.4 Adjustments and Modifications

If you find your calculated zones don't feel right:

Heart rate too high for perceived effort: Drop each zone by 5-10 bpm. POTS patients often have higher resting heart rates, which can throw off standard calculations.

Heart rate too low for perceived effort: Increase each zone by 5-10 bpm. Some medications or individual variations affect these calculations.

Use the talk test:

- Recovery/Base Pace: Should be able to speak in full sentences
- Maximal Steady State: Can speak short phrases, 3-4 words
- Intervals: Can barely speak, one word answers

Adjustments I've made to standard zones:

Why I made these adjustments:

Appendix B: Equipment Shopping Guide

You need equipment to complete this program. Here's what to buy, where to find it, and how much to budget.

B.1 Essential Equipment

Recumbent Cardio (need at least ONE):

Recumbent Bike

- Budget: $150-300 (basic models)
- Mid-range: $300-600 (better quality, more features)
- High-end: $600-1,500 (commercial quality)
- Recommended brands: Schwinn (270 model ~$500), Nautilus, Marcy
- Where to buy: Amazon, Dick's Sporting Goods, Walmart, local fitness stores
- Used options: Craigslist, Facebook Marketplace, Play It Again Sports
- What to look for: Adjustable seat, smooth pedaling, stable frame, heart rate monitor built-in (nice but not essential)

Supine Pedaler (Under Desk Bike)

- Budget: $30-80
- Best option if space limited or budget tight
- Recommended: DeskCycle ($150 but excellent quality), MagneTrainer, generic versions on Amazon
- Where to buy: Amazon, Target
- What to look for: Smooth resistance, stable base, fits under your bed or desk
- Limitation: Less resistance than recumbent bike, but works for Phase 1-2

Rowing Machine

- Budget: $200-400 (chain drive models)
- Mid-range: $400-800 (better resistance)
- High-end: $800-1,200 (Concept2, commercial quality)
- Recommended: Concept2 Model D (~$900, gold standard), Sunny Health & Fitness (budget)
- Where to buy: Rogue Fitness, Amazon, Dick's Sporting Goods
- What to look for: Smooth slide, comfortable seat, easy to get on/off
- Note: Works whole body, so monitor heart rate closely

Pool Access (Alternative)

- Cost: $30-80/month gym membership with pool
- Free: Community pools in summer, local recreation centers
- Best option if you have joint issues or heat intolerance
- Limitation: Requires access and travel

Strength Training Equipment:

Resistance Bands Set

- Cost: $10-30 for complete set
- Recommended: TheraBand sets, Fit Simplify, Black Mountain
- Where to buy: Amazon, Target, Walmart, sporting goods stores
- What to get: Set with multiple resistance levels (light, medium, heavy)
- Essential: Get set with handles and door anchor

Optional Additions:

- Yoga mat: $15-30 (for floor exercises)
- Small dumbbells: $20-50 for set of 3-8 lb pairs (for progression)
- Stability ball: $15-25 (for core work)

Heart Rate Monitor (Recommended):

Chest Strap Monitors

- Cost: $30-60
- Most accurate option
- Recommended: Polar H10 (~$90), Wahoo TICKR (~$50)
- Syncs with apps and equipment

Watch-Based Monitors

- Cost: $50-400
- Convenient but less accurate for POTS
- Options: Fitbit Charge (budget), Garmin Forerunner (mid-range), Apple Watch (high-end)
- Note: Wrist-based monitors can be inaccurate with POTS

Finger Pulse Oximeter

- Cost: $15-30
- Quick checks during exercise
- Not for continuous monitoring
- Budget-friendly option

B.2 Budget Packages

Bare Minimum Package ($40-110):

- Supine pedaler: $30-80
- Resistance band set: $10-30
- **Total: $40-110**
- Enough to complete Phase 1 and 2, transition to upright requires more options

Standard Package ($200-380):

- Recumbent bike (used or budget model): $150-300
- Resistance band set: $10-30
- Yoga mat: $15-25
- Chest strap HR monitor: $30-60 (optional but helpful)
- **Total: $200-380**
- Everything needed for full 16-week program

Optimal Package ($700-1,100):

- Quality recumbent bike: $500-800
- Resistance band set: $10-30
- Small dumbbell set: $40-80
- Yoga mat: $15-25
- Stability ball: $15-25
- Chest strap HR monitor: $50-90
- Foam roller: $20-40 (recovery)
- **Total: $700-1,100**
- Sets you up for long-term success

Gym Membership Alternative:

- Cost: $10-40/month ($120-480 for 12 months)
- Access to all equipment
- Option for pool
- Consider: Travel to gym, upright time walking around, crowding during peak hours
- Best if: Live close to gym with good equipment

B.3 Where to Find Used Equipment

Facebook Marketplace:

- Locally available, can test before buying
- Look for: Recumbent bikes, rowing machines
- Red flags: Wobbly, squeaky, rusted, major scratches suggest heavy wear
- Negotiate: Start at 50-60% of asking price
- Safety: Meet in public, bring someone with you

Craigslist:

- Similar to Facebook Marketplace
- More scams, be cautious
- Never send money before seeing item

Play It Again Sports:

- Used sporting goods stores
- Higher prices than private sellers but verified condition
- Can test in store
- Sometimes have warranties

Garage Sales / Estate Sales:

- Best deals possible
- Hit or miss on availability
- Bring cash
- Test before buying

Nextdoor App:

- Neighborhood-specific
- Often free items or cheap
- Building community connections

OfferUp / Letgo:

- Similar to Facebook Marketplace
- Rating systems for buyers/sellers

B.4 Equipment Alternatives

No Equipment at All:

- Supine leg cycling in bed (free, described in Chapter 4.0)
- Chair cardio (requires sturdy chair only)
- Bodyweight strength exercises
- Walking stairs in your home
- **Limitation**: Harder to progress intensity and track metrics

Travel / Minimal Space Solutions:

- Resistance bands (pack flat, travel anywhere)
- Supine pedaler (fits under bed)
- Bodyweight exercises
- Walk local stairs or paths
- Hotel gym access

B.5 Shopping Checklist

Before I start Week 1, I will have:

[ ] At least one recumbent cardio option: ____________________

[ ] Resistance bands or dumbbells: ____________________

[ ] Heart rate monitoring method: ____________________

[ ] Mat or comfortable floor surface: ____________________

[ ] Upright cardio option for Phase 3-4: ____________________

Equipment I already own:

____

____

Equipment I need to acquire:

____

____

My budget: $ __________

Where I'll shop:

Timeline for acquisition: By date: _________

Appendix C: Hydration and Electrolyte Recipes

POTS management requires high sodium and fluid intake. These recipes make it easier and more palatable. All recipes designed for daily use throughout the program.

C.1 Electrolyte Drink Recipes

Basic Electrolyte Drink (Simple, Budget-Friendly)

Ingredients:

- 16 oz water
- 1/4 tsp salt (600 mg sodium)
- Juice of 1/2 lemon or lime
- 1 tsp honey or sugar (optional, for taste)

Instructions: Mix thoroughly. Drink 30-60 minutes before exercise or throughout day.

Cost per serving: $0.10-0.25

Enhanced Electrolyte Drink (Better Taste, More Minerals)

Ingredients:

- 16 oz water
- 1/4 tsp salt (600 mg sodium)
- 1/4 tsp lite salt or salt substitute (potassium)
- Juice of 1/2 lemon
- 1 tsp honcy
- Pinch of magnesium powder (optional)

Instructions: Mix thoroughly. Best served cold over ice.

Cost per serving: $0.20-0.40

Orange Sports Drink (Commercial Taste)

Ingredients:

- 16 oz water
- 1/4 tsp salt (600 mg sodium)
- 2 tbsp orange juice concentrate
- 1 tsp sugar
- Tiny pinch of citric acid powder (optional, for tartness)

Instructions: Mix well, shake in bottle. Tastes similar to commercial sports drinks but with more sodium.

Cost per serving: $0.30-0.50

Coconut Water Base Drink

Ingredients:

- 8 oz coconut water (natural potassium)
- 8 oz water
- 1/4 tsp salt added (coconut water has minimal sodium)
- Squeeze of lime

Instructions: Mix well. Coconut water provides natural electrolytes but needs salt added.

Cost per serving: $0.75-1.25

C.2 High Sodium Meal Ideas

You need 10-12 grams of sodium daily. That's 10,000-12,000 mg. Here's how:

Breakfast Options (2,000-3,000 mg sodium):

Salty Oatmeal

- Instant oatmeal: 300 mg
- Add 1/4 tsp salt: +600 mg
- Add 1 oz cheese: +200 mg
- Side of 2 slices toast with salted butter: +400 mg
- Glass of V8 juice: +500 mg
- **Total: ~2,000 mg**

Eggs and Sausage

- 2 eggs scrambled with salt (1/4 tsp added): 750 mg

- 2 sausage links: 500 mg
- Hash browns with ketchup: 400 mg
- Glass of tomato juice: 500 mg
- **Total: ~2,150 mg**

Lunch Options (2,500-3,500 mg sodium):

Deli Sandwich

- 2 slices bread: 300 mg
- 4 oz deli meat (turkey, ham): 1,200-1,600 mg
- Cheese slice: 200 mg
- Mustard, pickles: 300 mg
- Side of chips (1 oz): 150 mg
- Side of pretzels (1 oz): 400 mg
- **Total: ~2,550-3,150 mg**

Canned Soup and Crackers

- 1 can Campbell's soup (condensed, prepared): 1,800-2,500 mg
- Saltine crackers (10): 300 mg
- Cheese (1 oz): 200 mg
- **Total: ~2,300-3,000 mg**

Dinner Options (2,500-4,000 mg sodium):

Pasta with Sauce

- Pasta (2 cups cooked): 0-10 mg (needs salt added)
- Add 1/2 tsp salt to cooking water: +1,200 mg
- Jarred pasta sauce (1 cup): 700-1,000 mg
- Parmesan cheese (2 tbsp): 200 mg
- Garlic bread (2 slices): 400 mg
- **Total: ~2,500-2,800 mg**

Stir Fry with Soy Sauce

- Chicken or tofu: minimal sodium
- Vegetables: minimal sodium
- 2 tbsp soy sauce: 1,800-2,000 mg
- Add 1/4 tsp salt: +600 mg
- Served over rice: 0 mg (add salt to rice water)
- **Total: ~2,400-3,200 mg**

Snack Options (500-1,500 mg each):

- Pretzels (2 oz): 800 mg
- Salted peanuts (2 oz): 300-600 mg
- Pickles (1 large): 1,200-1,500 mg
- Olives (10): 500-700 mg
- Popcorn with salt (3 cups): 600-800 mg
- String cheese (2): 400 mg
- Beef jerky (1 oz): 500-700 mg
- Saltines (20): 600 mg

C.3 Salt Loading Methods

Straight Salt (Fastest Method):

- 1/4 tsp salt = 600 mg sodium
- 1/2 tsp salt = 1,200 mg sodium
- 1 tsp salt = 2,400 mg sodium

How to take straight salt:

- Mix in 2-4 oz water, drink quickly
- Put on tongue, wash down with water
- Mix into applesauce
- Take before exercise or when feeling symptomatic

Salt tablets/capsules:

- Available at pharmacies and online
- Common: 1 gram (1,000 mg) sodium per tablet
- Easier to take than loose salt
- More expensive but convenient
- Take with full glass of water

Broth/Bouillon:

- 1 cup bouillon: 800-1,200 mg sodium
- Hot, soothing, hydrating
- Good morning option
- Easy on stomach
- Cheap and convenient

C.4 Daily Hydration Schedule

Sample schedule to reach 10 grams sodium and 2.5 liters fluid:

Morning (7:00 AM):

- 8 oz water with 1/4 tsp salt (600 mg)
- Or 1 cup bouillon (1,000 mg)

Breakfast (8:00 AM):

- Salty meal (2,000-3,000 mg sodium)
- 8 oz juice or water

Mid-Morning (10:30 AM):

- 16 oz electrolyte drink (600 mg sodium)

Before Exercise (30-60 min prior):

- 8-16 oz electrolyte drink (300-600 mg sodium)

During Exercise:

- Sip 4-8 oz water or electrolyte drink

Immediately After Exercise:

- 16-24 oz electrolyte drink with extra salt (600-1,200 mg sodium)

Lunch (12:30 PM):

- Salty meal (2,500-3,500 mg sodium)
- 8 oz water or diet soda

Afternoon (3:00 PM):

- 16 oz water
- Salty snack (500-1,000 mg sodium)

Dinner (6:00 PM):

- Salty meal (2,500-4,000 mg sodium)
- 8 oz water

Evening (8:00 PM):

- 8-16 oz water or herbal tea
- Salt tablet if needed to reach goal

Before Bed:

- 8 oz water

Total: ~10,000-12,000 mg sodium, 2.5-3 liters fluid

C.5 Tracking Template

Daily Sodium and Fluid Log

Date: __________

Sodium Goal: 10,000 mg **Fluid Goal:** 2,500 ml

Time	Food/Drink	Sodium (mg)	Fluid (oz)

Total Sodium: _____ mg **Total Fluid:** _____ oz (_____ ml)

Did I meet goals? [ ] Yes [ ] No

How I felt today: ____

Adjustments for tomorrow: ______________________________________

Appendix D: Sample Week Templates

Use these blank templates to plan upcoming weeks or customize the program for your needs.

D.1 Blank Weekly Overview

Week _____ Overview (Phase _____)

Date Range: __________ to __________

Goals for this week:

1. ______________________________
2. ______________________________
3. ______________________________

Cardio prescription:

- Duration: _____ to _____ minutes per session
- Intensity: ______________ zone(s)
- Position: [ ] Recumbent [ ] Upright [ ] Mixed
- Frequency: _____ sessions this week

Strength prescription:

- Sessions: _____ this week (which days: ____)
- Focus: ______________________________

Special considerations this week:

____

____

D.2 Blank Daily Exercise Log

Day: __________ Date: __________ Week: _____

Morning status:

- Sleep: _____ hours
- Resting HR: _____ bpm
- How I feel (1-10): _____
- Symptoms:

  ____

Cardio Session:

Equipment:

____

Planned duration: _____ minutes Actual duration: _____ minutes

Position: [ ] Recumbent [ ] Upright [ ] Mixed

Target zone: ________________ Actual HR: Start _____ Mid _____ End _____ Peak _____

RPE (1-10): _____

During exercise (1-10): _____

Symptoms during:

____

2-4 hours after (1-10): _____

Next morning (1-10): _____

Strength Session: [ ] Completed [ ] Skipped

Exercises done:

____

____

Notes:

____

____

____

What went well: ____

What to adjust: ____

D.3 Custom Week Designer

Use this to create your own modified weeks

My Custom Week for: (week number/situation) __________________________

Why I'm customizing: ____

Monday:

- Cardio: _____ min at ______________ intensity on __________________________
- Strength: [ ] Yes [ ] No Exercises: _______________________________________

Tuesday:

- Cardio: _____ min at ______________ intensity on __________________________
- Strength: [ ] Yes [ ] No Exercises: _______________________________________

Wednesday:

- Cardio: _____ min at ______________ intensity on __________________________
- Strength: [ ] Yes [ ] No Exercises: _______________________________________

Thursday:

- Cardio: _____ min at ______________ intensity on __________________________
- Strength: [ ] Yes [ ] No Exercises: _______________________________________

Friday:

- Cardio: _____ min at ______________ intensity on __________________________
- Strength: [ ] Yes [ ] No Exercises: _______________________________________

Saturday:

- Cardio: _____ min at ______________ intensity on __________________________
- Strength: [ ] Yes [ ] No Exercises: _______________________________________

Sunday:

- [ ] Rest day [ ] Light activity: ____

Total planned minutes this week: _____ minutes

Expected challenges: ____

____

How I'll address them: ____

____

Appendix E: Research References and Further Reading

The protocols in this workbook are based on established research. This appendix provides the key studies and resources for deeper understanding.

E.1 Core Research Studies

Foundational POTS Exercise Research:

Fu, Q., & Levine, B. D. (2018). Exercise and non-pharmacological treatment of POTS. Autonomic Neuroscience, 215, 20-27. https://doi.org/10.1016/j.autneu.2018.07.001

George, S. A., Bivens, T. B., Howden, E. J., Saleem, Y., Galbreath, M. M., Hendrickson, D., Fu, Q., & Levine, B. D. (2016). The international POTS registry: Evaluating the efficacy of an exercise training intervention in a community setting. Heart Rhythm, 13(4), 943-950. https://doi.org/10.1016/j.hrthm.2015.12.012

Shibata, S., Fu, Q., Bivens, T. B., Hastings, J. L., Wang, W., & Levine, B. D. (2012). Short-term exercise training improves the cardiovascular response to exercise in the postural orthostatic tachycardia syndrome. The Journal of Physiology, 590(15), 3495-3505. https://doi.org/10.1113/jphysiol.2012.233858

Clinical Protocols:

Levine Exercise Protocol (original publication): Fu, Q., VanGundy, T. B., Shibata, S., Auchus, R. J., Williams, G. H., & Levine, B. D. (2011). Exercise training versus propranolol in the treatment of the postural orthostatic tachycardia syndrome. Hypertension, 58(2), 167-175. https://doi.org/10.1161/HYPERTENSIONAHA.111.172262

Children's Hospital of Philadelphia (CHOP) Protocol information available at: https://www.chop.edu/conditions-diseases/postural-orthostatic-tachycardia-syndrome-pots

POTS Pathophysiology:

Raj, S. R., Guzman, J. C., Harvey, P., Richer, L., Schondorf, R., Seifer, C., Thibodeau-Jarry, N., Sheldon, R. S., & POTS Calgary-Niagara Investigators. (2020). Canadian Cardiovascular Society position statement on postural orthostatic tachycardia syndrome (POTS) and related disorders of chronic orthostatic intolerance. Canadian Journal of Cardiology, 36(3), 357-372. https://doi.org/10.1016/j.cjca.2019.12.024

Sheldon, R. S., Grubb, B. P., Olshansky, B., Shen, W. K., Calkins, H., Brignole, M., Raj, S. R., Krahn, A. D., Morillo, C. A., Stewart, J. M., Sutton, R., Sandroni, P., Friday, K. J., Hachul, D. T., Cohen, M. I., Lau, D. H., Mayuga, K. A., Moak, J. P., Sandhu, R. K., & Kanjwal, K. (2015). 2015 Heart Rhythm Society expert consensus statement on the diagnosis and treatment of postural tachycardia syndrome, inappropriate sinus tachycardia, and vasovagal syncope. Heart Rhythm, 12(6), e41-e63. https://doi.org/10.1016/j.hrthm.2015.03.029

E.2 Books and Clinical Guides

For Patients:

"POTS: Together We Stand" by Lauren Stiles and the Dysautonomia International Medical Advisory Board

- Comprehensive patient guide to POTS management
- Includes exercise protocols and lifestyle modifications

"The Dysautonomia Project: Understanding Autonomic Nervous System Disorders for Patients and Caregivers" by Kelly Freeman, PhD and Anthony Goodman, MD

- Detailed explanation of dysautonomia conditions including POTS
- Treatment approaches and research updates

For Clinicians:

"Primer on the Autonomic Nervous System" (Third Edition) edited by Phillip A. Low and Eduardo E. Benarroch

- Academic textbook covering autonomic dysfunction
- Technical depth for healthcare providers

E.3 Online Resources

Dysautonomia International Website: www.dysautonomiainternational.org

- Patient advocacy organization
- Research updates and clinical resources
- Physician directory

- Support groups

Standing Up to POTS Website: www.standinguptopots.org

- Patient education and advocacy
- Exercise resources and support
- Community forums

National Institutes of Health (NIH) Genetic and Rare Diseases Information Center: https://rarediseases.info.nih.gov/diseases/9597/postural-orthostatic-tachycardia-syndrome

- Medical information and research updates

Bateman Horne Center Website: www.batemanhornecenter.org

- Clinical research center for complex chronic illnesses
- POTS education and resources

E.4 Research on Comorbidities

POTS and EDS:

Hakim, A., O'Callaghan, C., De Wandele, I., Stiles, L., Pocinki, A., & Rowe, P. (2017). Cardiovascular autonomic dysfunction in Ehlers-Danlos syndrome—Hypermobile type. American Journal of Medical Genetics Part C: Seminars in Medical Genetics, 175(1), 168-174. https://doi.org/10.1002/ajmg.c.31543

POTS and MCAS:

Mast cell activation may complicate POTS management. Coordination with specialist important for patients with both conditions.

POTS and ME/CFS:

Exercise intolerance patterns differ. Patients with both conditions may need more conservative approach.

E.5 For Healthcare Providers

Clinical Assessment Tools:

Autonomic testing (tilt table, active stand test) available through specialized autonomic laboratories.

Mayo Clinic Autonomic Reflex Screen standardized assessment battery.

Treatment Guidelines:

2015 Heart Rhythm Society Expert Consensus Statement (cited above in E.1) provides comprehensive clinical guidelines for POTS diagnosis and treatment.

Continuing Education:

American Autonomic Society: www.americanautonomicsociety.org

- Annual conference and educational resources

Dysautonomia International Medical Webinar Series

- Regular webinars for healthcare providers

Appendix F: Printable Quick Reference Cards

Cut out these cards and keep them with your exercise equipment, in your workout bag, or posted where you'll see them daily.

F.1 Heart Rate Zone Card

MY HEART RATE ZONES

Age: _____ Max HR: _____ bpm

RECOVERY ZONE (50-60%)
_____ to _____ bpm | RPE 3-4
Use in: Phase 1, warm-ups, recovery days

BASE PACE ZONE (60-70%)
_____ to _____ bpm | RPE 5-6
Use in: Phase 1-2, steady state sessions

MAXIMAL STEADY STATE (70-80%)
_____ to _____ bpm | RPE 7-8
Use in: Phase 2-3, harder sessions

INTERVAL ZONE (80-90%)
_____ to _____ bpm | RPE 9-10
Use in: Phase 4 only, brief intervals

F.2 Phase Prescription Card

16-WEEK PROGRAM PHASES

PHASE 1: Weeks 1-4
Position: All recumbent
Duration: 3-20 minutes
Intensity: Recovery to Base Pace
Frequency: 5-6 days/week

PHASE 2: Weeks 5-8
Position: All recumbent
Duration: 20-30 minutes
Intensity: Base Pace to Maximal Steady State
Frequency: 5-6 days/week

PHASE 3: Weeks 9-12
Position: Begin upright (Weeks 10-12)
Duration: 25-35 minutes
Intensity: Base Pace to Maximal Steady State
Frequency: 5-6 days/week

PHASE 4: Weeks 13-16
Position: Primarily upright
Duration: 30-45 minutes
Intensity: Full range including intervals
Frequency: 5-6 days/week

F.3 Pre-Exercise Checklist Card

BEFORE EVERY SESSION

□ Hydrated (8-16 oz fluid 30-60 min ago)

□ Extra sodium consumed (if needed)

□ Compression garments on (if prescribed)

□ At least 5 hours sleep last night

□ Not actively fighting infection/illness

□ No fever or chest pain

□ HR monitor ready (if using)

□ Water bottle nearby

□ Know today's prescription:
Duration: _____ min
Intensity: ___________
Position: ___________

IF ANY RED FLAGS, SKIP OR MODIFY TODAY

F.4 Stop Exercise Immediately Card

STOP EXERCISE IF:

- Chest pain or pressure
- Irregular heartbeat
- Severe dizziness or near-fainting
- Vision changes (seeing spots, blackout)
- Severe nausea
- Extreme shortness of breath
- Feeling of impending doom
- Unable to maintain balance

AFTER STOPPING:
→ Sit or lie down immediately
→ Check heart rate if possible
→ Drink fluids with sodium
→ Stay down 15-30 minutes
→ Call doctor if symptoms don't resolve

RESUME EXERCISE:
Only when symptoms back to baseline
AND after 1-2 good days

F.5 Daily Hydration and Sodium Card

DAILY TARGETS

SODIUM: 10,000-12,000 mg (10-12 grams)
□ Morning: 2,000-3,000 mg
□ Lunch: 2,500-3,500 mg
□ Dinner: 2,500-4,000 mg
□ Snacks: 1,000-2,000 mg
□ Before exercise: 300-600 mg

FLUID: 2.5-3 liters (80-100 oz)
□ Morning: 16 oz
□ Before exercise: 8-16 oz
□ After exercise: 16-24 oz
□ Throughout day: 40-60 oz

TIMING:

• Front-load before exercise
• Extra salt 30 min before session
• Drink immediately after exercise
• Spread throughout day

F.6 Crash Recovery Card

IF YOU CRASH

IMMEDIATE ACTIONS:
1. Complete rest 24-48 hours minimum
2. Increase sodium and fluids
3. Stay horizontal as much as possible
4. Sleep as much as body wants
5. Don't panic—this is recoverable

RESUMING EXERCISE:

Mild crash (symptoms 20-30% worse):
→ 1-2 days off
→ Resume at previous week's level

Moderate crash (symptoms 50%+ worse):
→ 3-4 days off
→ Drop back one full week

Severe crash (back to baseline):
→ Full week off minimum
→ Restart at Week 1
→ Investigate cause thoroughly

READY TO RESUME WHEN:
✓ Symptoms back to baseline
✓ Two consecutive good days
✓ Adequate sleep
✓ Not fighting illness

Appendix G: Working with Healthcare Providers

Use these templates to share your progress with your medical team. Organized documentation helps them support your reconditioning efforts.

G.1 Initial Exercise Clearance Form

POTS Exercise Reconditioning Program - Medical Clearance Request

Patient Name: ____

Date: __________

Dear Dr. ________________________,

I am beginning a 16-week cardiovascular reconditioning program specifically designed for POTS patients. This program is based on the Levine and CHOP exercise protocols, which research has shown improve POTS symptoms in 60-90% of patients who complete them.

The program:

- Starts with 3-5 minutes of recumbent exercise
- Builds gradually over 16 weeks to 30-45 minutes
- Remains recumbent for first 8-9 weeks
- Introduces upright exercise gradually in weeks 10-12
- Uses heart rate monitoring to prevent overexertion

I am requesting your clearance to participate in this program.

My current medications:

____

____

____

My current POTS symptoms:

____

Specific concerns you should know about:

Questions for you:

1. Are there any medical reasons I should not participate?

2. Should I modify the program based on my medications or comorbidities?

3. What symptoms should prompt me to stop and contact you?

4. How often should I check in with you during the program?

Physician Approval:

□ I approve participation in this exercise reconditioning program as described.

□ I approve with the following modifications: ______________________________

□ I do not approve participation due to: __________________________________

Physician Signature: ___________________________ Date: __________

G.2 Monthly Progress Report Template

POTS Exercise Program - Month _____ Update

Patient Name: _______________________________ **Date:** __________

Program Status: Completed Week _____ of 16 (Phase _____)

Exercise Completion:

- Sessions completed: _____ out of _____ prescribed
- Completion rate: _____%
- Current duration: _____ minutes per session
- Current intensity: _________________ heart rate zone

Symptom Changes:

Improved:

Unchanged:

Worsened:

Cardiovascular Measurements:

Metric	Baseline	Current	Change
Resting HR (lying)	_____	_____	_____
Standing HR (1 min)	_____	_____	_____
Standing HR (3 min)	_____	_____	_____
Standing tolerance	_____ min	_____ min	_____
Orthostatic increase	_____ bpm	_____ bpm	_____

Functional Improvements:

Activities I can now do that I couldn't do before:

Challenges Encountered:

Modifications Made:

Questions for Provider:

1.
2.
3.

Medication Changes Needed?

Next Steps:

G.3 Completion Report Template

POTS Exercise Program - 16-Week Completion Report

Patient Name: ________________________________ **Date:** __________

Program Status: □ Completed all 16 weeks □ Completed _____ weeks

Overall Completion:

- Total sessions: _____ out of 96 prescribed cardio sessions
- Completion rate: _____%
- Final session capacity: _____ minutes at __________ intensity

Symptom Outcomes:

Significantly Improved:

____

____

Moderately Improved:

____

____

Unchanged:

____

Worsened:

____

Cardiovascular Outcomes:

Metric	Baseline	Post-Program	Change	% Change
Resting HR (lying)	_____	_____	_____	_____%
Standing HR (1 min)	_____	_____	_____	_____%
Standing HR (3 min)	_____	_____	_____	_____%
Standing tolerance	_____ min	_____ min	_____	_____%
Orthostatic increase	_____ bpm	_____ bpm	_____	_____%

Functional Outcomes:

Activities I can now do:

1. ______________________________
2. ______________________________
3. ______________________________
4. ______________________________
5. ______________________________

Quality of Life Impact:

Overall improvement rating (1-10, where 10=dramatically better): _____

How this program changed my life:

____

____

____

____

Maintenance Plan:

Exercise frequency moving forward: _____ days per week

Duration per session: _____ minutes

Planned activities:

____

____

Recommendations:

What worked best for me:

____

____

What I would modify:

____

____

Provider Follow-Up Needed:

□ Medication adjustments based on improvement

□ Continued monitoring (frequency: _____________)

□ Additional testing or assessment

□ Referral to: ____

□ No changes needed at this time

Patient Signature: ______________________________ **Date:** __________

Provider Signature: ______________________________ **Date:** __________

Reference

- Fu, Q., & Levine, B. D. (2018). Exercise and non-pharmacological treatment of POTS. *Autonomic Neuroscience: Basic and Clinical, 215*, 20–27. doi:10.1016/j.autneu.2018.07.001
- George, S. A., Bivens, T. B., Howden, E. J., Saleem, Y., Galbreath, M. M., Hendrickson, D., Fu, Q., & Levine, B. D. (2016). The international POTS registry: Evaluating the efficacy of an exercise training intervention in a community setting. *Heart Rhythm, 13*(4), 943–950. doi:10.1016/j.hrthm.2015.12.012
- Raj, S. R., Guzman, J. C., Harvey, P., Richer, L., Schondorf, R., Seifer, C., Thibodeau-Jarry, N., Sheldon, R. S., & CCS POTS Guideline Panel. (2020). Canadian Cardiovascular Society position statement on postural orthostatic tachycardia syndrome (POTS) and related disorders of chronic orthostatic intolerance. *Canadian Journal of Cardiology, 36*(3), 357–372. doi:10.1016/j.cjca.2019.12.024
- Sheldon, R. S., Grubb, B. P., Olshansky, B., Shen, W.-K., Calkins, H., Brignole, M., Raj, S. R., Krahn, A. D., Morillo, C. A., Stewart, J. M., Sutton, R., Sandroni, P., Friday, K. J., Hachul, D. T., Cohen, M. I., Lau, D. H., Mayuga, K. A., Moak, J. P., Sandhu, R. K., & Kanjwal, K. (2015). 2015 Heart Rhythm Society expert consensus statement on the diagnosis and treatment of postural tachycardia syndrome, inappropriate sinus tachycardia, and vasovagal syncope. *Heart Rhythm, 12*(6), e41–e63. doi:10.1016/j.hrthm.2015.03.029
- Shibata, S., Fu, Q., Bivens, T. B., Hastings, J. L., Wang, W., & Levine, B. D. (2012). Short-term exercise training improves the cardiovascular response to exercise in the postural orthostatic tachycardia syndrome. *The Journal of Physiology, 590*(15), 3495–3505. doi:10.1113/jphysiol.2012.233858

Made in the USA
Monee, IL
15 September 2026

63194582R00138